the way of the fertile soul

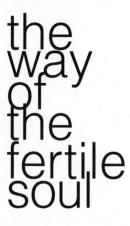

the way of the fertile soul

Ten Ancient Chinese
Secrets to Tap
into a Woman's
Creative Potential

Randine Lewis, Ph.D., L.Ac.

ATRIA BOOKS
New York London Toronto Sydney

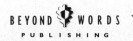
BEYOND WORDS
PUBLISHING

ATRIA BOOKS
A Division of Simon & Schuster, Inc.
1230 Avenue of the Americas
New York, NY 10020

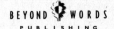BEYOND WORDS
PUBLISHING
20827 N.W. Cornell Road, Suite 500
Hillsboro, Oregon 97124-9808

The information contained in this book is intended to be educational and not for diagnosis, prescription, or treatment of any health disorder whatsoever. This information should not replace consultation with a competent health care professional. The content of the book is intended to be used as an adjunct to a rational and responsible health care program prescribed by a professional health care practitioner. The author and publisher are in no way liable for any misuse of the material.

Editor: Jenefer Angell
Managing editor: Lindsay S. Brown
Copyeditor: Toby Yuen
Proofreader: Meadowlark Communications, Inc.
Cover & interior design: Carol Sibley and Sara E. Blum
Compositions: William H. Brunson Typography Services

First Atria Books/Beyond Words trade paperback edition November 2007

Manufactured in the United States of America

ISBN-13: 978-1-58270-180-6

This book is dedicated to my parents,
Diane Ellison and Brooks Anderson,
from whom I learned unconditional love.

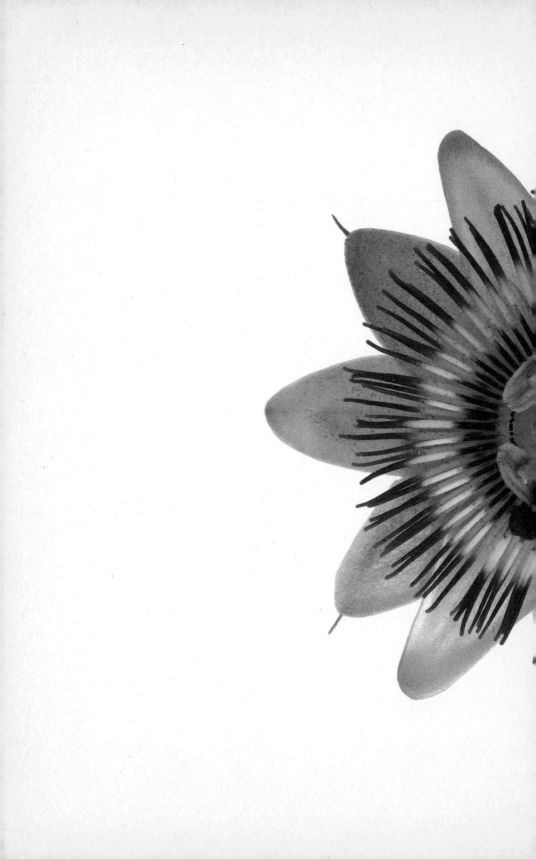

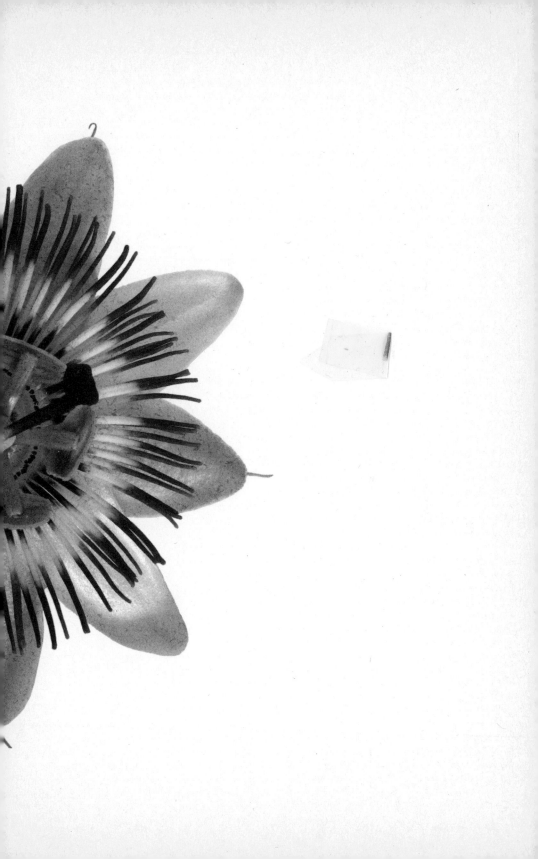

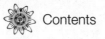 Contents

Acknowledgments

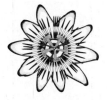

I would like to extend my unending gratitude to the Mysterious Mother, whom I will never understand but will always revere. When I become too full of myself, she pulls me back into the lap of her fierce reality, and helps me return to my truth, which is hers. I thank her for the many difficult and wondrous opportunities for growth that have allowed me to surrender to her wisdom. She has taken many forms—my own mother and grandmothers, and the mothers of the heart who make a difference in the world. A special thanks to my agent, Carol Susan Roth, and my publisher, Cynthia Black, who believed in the message I have to convey. I would also like to recognize the amazing Fertile Soul staff, and the practitioners of The Fertile Soul clinics who help facilitate the remedy for today's healing crisis. I would also like to thank those who have taken the courage to reach out for help, and those who have discovered that true healing must come from within, as they give birth to their real selves. May you continue to be restored as you dip into the unfathomable depth of the well of the Mysterious Mother. Come, drink; you need never thirst again.

Preface

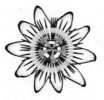

The idea to write this book grew out of my desire to expand the concept of women's fertility. When I told my patients that I was going to write *The Way of the Fertile Soul*, they urged me to share what they had learned about the real soul of Chinese medicine and meditation.

I help women conceive. But more than that, I help them give birth to the deepest part of themselves, whether they are trying to bring in a child or are looking for freedom in any aspect of their life—at any age. This book is meant to bridge the gap between the full meaning of fertility and the narrow definition it has been limited to. *The Way of the Fertile Soul* is intended to open you up to create life in its myriad forms. Whether or not you are seeking to bear a child, this process is a tool to help you open up to the fruitfulness at your very core. Those trying to have a baby find that it opens them up to the life-giving powers of the universe.

In the present time, as women redefine themselves once again, we are pregnant with possibility, ready to give birth to our own liberation. Fertility is life.

Introduction:
Living the Life You Want

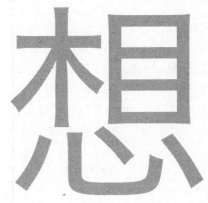

想 *Hope*

You are indeed carrying within yourself the potential to visualize, to design, and to create an utterly satisfying, joyful, and pure lifestyle.

— RAINER MARIA RILKE

When I began, more than twenty years ago, to research a successful infertility cure, I looked to ancient sources of Eastern wisdom: the Tao and traditional Chinese medicine. These systems have helped people around the globe create inner balance and live in harmony with their environment for thousands of years; I reinterpreted their guidance to apply to women in the twenty-first century. I uncovered ten secrets and developed a program that enables women who previously couldn't conceive to become pregnant and have healthy babies.

At first, I taught my technique only to help women become pregnant, and my program resulted in an astonishing increase in participants' pregnancy rate. But I also found that it resulted in helping women move forward and feel increased vitality and contentment in all areas of their lives, from their work to their home life to their sense of self. As their fierce fight to have a child lessened, the women found that they were more capable of living a calm yet energized happy life and they were able to more easily fulfill their most cherished dreams. Letting go instead of resisting the way things are proved to be the path to serenity.

How can my program not only enable conception but reduce stress and increase vitality? It's because infertility, lack of vitality, and stress are bound together. They are all symptoms of a life out of balance. Our procreative energies are at the very core of our being and, if obstructed, can't be fully expressed. But once stress and the blocked energy, bodily imbalances, and dysfunctional organ responses it produces are released, women become not only more able to conceive but more relaxed, more receptive, and more joyful, open to new ideas, new projects, and new lives.

I've seen it time and time again. Rebecca, a psychotherapist who attended four of my Fertile Soul retreats, described how the ancient secrets helped her stop trying to force her destiny and live instead according to her true nature:

> It's like losing your keys. You look everywhere and anywhere—sometimes you look in the same place multiple times—but you still have no keys. It is when you give up looking that they suddenly appear under your nose and you're amazed that they were right

there the whole time. You swear you looked there! I looked for my keys (to a happier life) for three years. I used every flashlight, strobe light, and digging machine I could find. I didn't want to stop looking because I didn't want to give up that sense of control. Letting go of control is the hardest step of this program but it's the one with the greatest reward. When you stop trying to control the outcome, everything that you're looking for will come to you. Your keys will be found. They've been there all along.

My Personal Path to Balance

I discovered the ten secrets that let women reduce their stress and tap into the creative power of the universe when I was trying to prove myself to the world. In my twenties I became obsessed with my weight, my appearance, and my achievements. I developed addictive qualities and became more and more aware of the emptiness inside that I was desperately trying to fill with external pursuits, including the fight to have a child. Although I had conceived my first daughter fairly easily, things were much more difficult the second time around. I was fresh out of medical school, married to a physician, and determined to have another child. Month after month passed by without producing the longed-for result, and I became more and more obsessed with bearing another child.

I also started experiencing some unsettling hormonal problems. My periods became irregular, sometimes disappearing completely, my hair began to fall out, and I suffered through night sweats and joint pain. A visit to my gynecologist revealed I had extremely low estrogen and progesterone levels, which were preventing me from conceiving. My doctor recommended

I take a drug called Clomid (clomiphene citrate) to stimulate my ovaries to produce more eggs.

Though I was desperate enough to undergo just about any medical treatment to become pregnant, I decided against taking Clomid. I believed I had a problem with my entire hormonal system, not with egg production, and hormones couldn't rectify that. (I didn't know it then, but hormones operate via negative feedback, meaning that when you supply hormonal drugs from the outside, they shut off your body's own hormonal production.) My husband, Ed, also reminded me of the many medical problems that can result from hormonal stimulation. Deep within me I knew that a child wouldn't come simply because I demanded it.

So I decided to heal myself—the decision was the beginning of the end of my struggle. Somehow I knew that the only way I would really heal was from within. I read everything I could about conception and reproduction. I changed my lifestyle to include a more balanced eating plan and meditative movement exercises. Eventually, I stopped smoking, drinking alcohol, coffee, and diet soda, and eating milk products, sugar, and animal products. I drank wheatgrass every day and took several nutritional supplements. In other words, I took better care of myself.

Then I read a book that described how acupuncture could help treat infertility. So I started going to three different acupuncturists, who treated me in three different ways. I also began taking Chinese herbal fertility tonics, which smelled and tasted awful. I tried every possibility I came across. But as I chased more cures, I still didn't become pregnant.

My health improved enormously, though. My hair stopped falling out, the night sweats came less often, and my energy increased significantly. I felt like a stronger, healthier person, which allowed me to become even more comfortable with my new way of life. Soon I was actually enjoying life again—and became pregnant. I was thrilled—and hooked on the benefits of Oriental medicine.

To learn more about it, I enrolled in Chinese medical school at night and completed the four-year program in half that time. Then, to apply my new knowledge, I moved with my family to Dalian, China, to work in a hospital that treated patients exclusively with traditional Chinese medicine. After my return, I established a clinic in Houston, Texas, and began treating women with reproductive disorders. I also earned a Ph.D. in alternative medicine; my dissertation dealt with enhancing fertility using traditional Chinese medicine.

It was while I was in China that I first studied the ancient Chinese texts of the Tao and traditional Chinese medicine. I read about how Taoism, one of the most ancient ways of life, often called "The Way," promotes inner harmony by bringing energy sources into balance. And I researched the 5,000-year-old principles of traditional Chinese medicine, in which the body is understood through a holistic view of nature. As I worked at the Dalian hospital, and later when I returned to the United States, I saw firsthand the powerful results of applying those concepts and principles and started to use them in conjunction with Western medicine.

But my own struggles with reproduction weren't over. A few years after our second daughter was born, Ed and I decided to expand our family again. I became pregnant, but ten weeks into the pregnancy, I miscarried. I was inconsolable. I felt numb and deeply distressed, both physically and mentally.

But I continued to take care of my health—body, mind, and spirit. And after just a few months, I discovered that I was pregnant again.

But this pregnancy did not go easily. Early on, my hormone levels dropped, and I and everyone around me thought I would lose this baby, too. But instead of struggling and resisting the potential catastrophe, I followed what I had learned through studying the Tao: I surrendered. The possibility of losing another baby profoundly shifted my outlook on life and caused me to let go of the outcome.

That doesn't mean that everything went smoothly from that moment on—there were complications right up to the end. But because I let go of the outcome, I was able to feel a deep sense of serenity throughout that long and difficult experience, a peace that spread to every part of life. I also came to understand even more deeply how important it is for women to take charge of their health, nourish and care for their bodies, and release their stress no matter what they do in their everyday lives or which phase of life they're in. That understanding made me turn again to the ancient wisdom of the Tao and traditional Chinese medicine.

This time as I read the books, I realized that their principles had been determined and were supported by a male- or yang-dominated society and that the feminine, or yin, side of the teachings was hidden, untranslated, and ignored. I found new meaning in the old principles and saw that women needed to restore the balance of yin and yang by aligning the energies of their bodies, minds, and spirits. I found the feminine roots of the Tao and traditional Chinese medicine, which led me to develop a feminine model of balanced, fruitful living. This new model not only helps women conceive and deliver healthy babies but reduces stress and enables them to live comfortably, creatively, and fully throughout their lives.

The program is based on the ten secrets of healthful living that I discovered in the ancient tomes:

Secret 1:
Balance your energies—
physical, emotional, and spiritual.

和 *Harmony*

Secret 2:
Let yourself be who you are.

意 *Contentment*

Secret 3:
Find and embrace your inner spaciousness.

敞 *Openness*

Secret 4:
Allow life to live through you.

性 *Nature's Way*

Secret 5:
Let go of resistance.

撒 *Release*

Secret 6:
Live from your joy
rather than your fear.

生 *Emergence*

Secret 7:
Use your emotions to revitalize your life.

信 *Trust Your Emotions*

Secret 8:
Live "vertically" instead of "horizontally."
竖 *Alignment*

Secret 9:
Reenergize yourself by repatterning.
氣 *Vitality*

Secret 10:
Match your external actions to your internal blueprint.
行 *Embodiment*

The Way of the Fertile Soul details each of these powerful secrets and shows you how to use them to reduce stress, renew energy, and achieve the inner balance and harmony you need to fulfill all your cherished dreams. It also offers easy-to-understand information about the Tao and traditional Chinese medicine and provides you with exercises and other tools to help you discover and assess your own sources of imbalance and blocked energy. In addition, you'll hear how women who attended my Fertile Soul retreats around the world have used the ten secrets to revitalize and enrich their lives to an extent they hadn't thought possible. Michelle, who now works for The Fertile Soul organization, described her process this way:

> *I now feel that I have given birth to myself. I have struggled, but I have learned to nurture myself. Though the initial nurturing was more of a licking of*

*wounds, over time I began to fertilize my inner life—
my own fertile ground. With patience and fortitude,
new life sprouted, and by watering those delicate
ferns I have allowed myself to grow strong and fertile
in the life I was already living.*

Being fertile and fruitful doesn't apply only to giving birth to
a child. It also applies to giving birth to the self you want to be
and to a life filled with passion, strength, joy, and adventure. By
tapping into the power of the universe, from which all life—
babies, new ideas, new dreams, and new ways of being—arises
and by using the ten ancient secrets, you can reconnect with
your true nature and create a deeply satisfying way of living—
calm, vital, fruitful, and blissful.

*The Tao is called the Great Mother:
Empty yet inexhaustible,
It gives birth to infinite worlds.
It is always present within you.
You can use it any way you want.*

—Tao Te Ching

Part I

Three Sources of
Wisdom:
The Tao,
Traditional Chinese
Medicine,
and You

1

Using Ancient Wisdom to Improve Your Well-being:
A Primer to the Tao and Traditional Chinese Medicine

道 *The Way*

Just imagine what would happen if practicing physicians, the ones who come into contact directly with suffering humanity, had some acquaintance with Eastern systems of healing. The Spirit of the East surges through every pore as a balm for all the afflictions.

— CARL JUNG

The Tao Te Ching

The Tao simply means The Way. It is not a religion or a belief. It is a deep understanding that comes from viewing the natural processes of life on our planet: the way a flower blooms, the way an acorn bursts from a seed to become a towering oak tree, the way we all begin life as the pure potential of an embryo, full of our parents' hopes and desires for us and the promise created

3

with our first breath. The Tao describes a way of living that expands and deepens all the things that happen between our first breath and our last: what we do while we are on this planet, who we spend our time with, and how we take care of the precious life we were given.

The Chinese character for Tao incorporates the concept of the deepest part of our being, in alignment with the highest part of our selves. The ancients tapped into this deep awareness and alignment, which allowed them to view themselves as an integral part of the great whole. When we, too, tap into that understanding, we see that we are a microcosm of the universal forces of nature, that there is something more than ourselves. When we follow The Way, we become creation itself—something new, the fulfillment of a dream—and we abide by the same principles of physics that govern all natural things.

Taoists look at life as the miraculous intermingling of body, mind, and spirit. They believe that your body came into existence through forces beyond your control, and that your spirit— the enlivening force in everything that exists—entered the cells your parents comingled to produce your form. While your body develops according to the DNA patterning that was encoded in your embryonic cells, Taoists believe each person chooses how he or she will blossom. They believe that spirit enables us to blossom in many ways, and lets us choose which, if any, fruit we want to bear. And while our body's potential eventually is exhausted and, like autumn leaves that have fallen, our form begins to crumble, our spirit lives on in what we have created.

The Tao is the spiritual force that brings all of existence out of the void. You may want to think of it as an intelligent, creative power that caused time, form, and space to rise up when nothing in our world existed. This creative power has two polar charges: one positive, called yang, and one negative, called yin. Both are found throughout the cosmos, in all of nature, and in each of our cells.

From the Tao comes light energy that forms a network of existence. In human form this energy aligns itself horizontally and vertically. The horizontal lines determine the time/space plane that we know as our material life. The vertical lines determine our ability to ascend from lower to higher spiritual planes. The soul—which zips the spirit into material form, enabling it to manifest—arises from this "energy grid" and is integrated with the body, giving us our potential.

Though you may not think so at this point, every one of us— including you—has constant access to this potential, to the power of creation. To reach it, one turns attention within, becomes still, and merges with the limitless void each of us has in the center of our heart. When you do this you will see that you are connected to all of creation—to energy, possibilities, acceptance, and fruitfulness. As Lao Tzu, the sixth-century BC philosopher who is thought of as the founder of Taoism, wrote:

We join spokes together in a wheel,
but it is the center hole that makes the wagon move.
We shape clay into a pot,
but it is the emptiness inside that holds whatever we desire.
We hammer wood for a house,
but it is the inner space that makes it livable.
We work with being,
but nonbeing is what we use.

When we are born, we begin to grow into a predetermined horizontal plane of existence. But we also have within us a spark of the Divine—some call this God, spirit, harmony, or love, whatever feels right to you—that gives us our purpose, that lets us produce and create and manifest our dreams. If we can recognize and stay connected to this spark, it will guide us upward from our pure potential to our highest calling and show us our infinite possibilities.

The creative spark within all women I call the Divine feminine potential, or "Mysterious Mother," and I consider all women fertile souls who can recognize that spark and, through it, live happily according to The Way. Though Divine connection is and has always been accessible to all, over time many of us have become disconnected: our feet bound, our hands tied, and our souls stifled under various patriarchal systems. When we stop paying attention to our spark, we eventually lose power, and become stressed, depressed, and exhausted. This book will help to strengthen that connection again, help you open your eyes, your heart, and your life to its great potential. In the words of the Indian saint Amma Chi: "The essence of motherhood is not restricted to women who have given birth; it is a principle inherent in both women and men. It is an attitude of the mind. It is love—and that love is the very breath of life."

But how exactly do we open ourselves to our potential? How can we get back on the path we slipped off when we shed our childhood innocence? If you've ever thought that life would be easier and better if only you had a road map, you can take heart, because nature did provide you with one that you can easily learn to follow. All you need to do is to follow your natural tendencies—they will lead you to where you want to go.

First, however, you must open up to receiving your new path. As we learn in the story of the Zen master who could not teach a scholar because the scholar was too full of ideas, learning to empty yourself of forced ways of being will allow you to embrace your inner spaciousness and open your mind to a healthier and more vital approach to life.

Traditional Chinese Medicine

Chinese medicine views human beings as microcosms of the universe. Human brains contain about as many neurons and human bodies about the same number of cells as there are stars in our galaxy. The electrons within our cells orbit protons the way the Earth circles the sun, and at the same speed. And we breathe the air that has been breathed by every person and animal that has ever lived—Gandhi, Mary Magdalene, and pterodactyls.

According to Chinese medicine, everything in nature, including people, is composed of one energy or life force, called *qi* (pronounced "chee"). Like electricity, this energy aligns itself according to negative and positive polarities known as yin and yang and exists on three levels: source, soul, and spirit. People also live according to the changes of the four seasons, exhibit five energetic tendencies, follow six directions, and have eight primary modes of interaction based on the energies found in nature. When all of these systems are in balance, we exhibit a state of harmonious, high-quality energy that enables us to function at a higher level as well. When we are in balance, we are healthy, with vitality flowing unobstructed through our body, mind, and spirit.

The Three Levels of Energy

Some practitioners of Eastern healing believe that life is lived in a kind of upward-lifting spiral that follows the grid of horizontal and vertical energy I just described. Our lower energies, or pure potential, are at the bottom, the source level; and our highest energies, or spirit, are at the top. In the middle is the soul level, in which we interact with the world. Our aim throughout life is to move from the lowest level to the highest.

We live at the source or "essence" level—the foundation or energy spring—during the first phase of our life. During that time we connect with our potential and live centered on ourselves. You only have to look at a newborn baby to see this: she stays tightly coiled, her arms and legs pulled in, her hands clenched, gripping any finger with which they come in contact; she is comfortable when she is swaddled, just as she was when she was enclosed within the uterus. Once she emerges, she lives according to her genetic imprint, and as she contin-

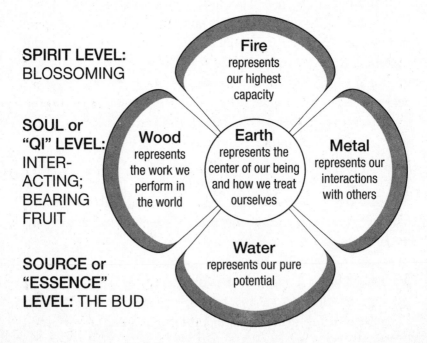

SPIRIT LEVEL: BLOSSOMING

SOUL or "QI" LEVEL: INTER-ACTING; BEARING FRUIT

SOURCE or "ESSENCE" LEVEL: THE BUD

Fire represents our highest capacity

Wood represents the work we perform in the world

Earth represents the center of our being and how we treat ourselves

Metal represents our interactions with others

Water represents our pure potential

ues to follow that blueprint she layers on top of it what her life will become.

Research in quantum physics has shown that our beliefs actually reinforce and reshape the very structure of our DNA. In his book *The Biology of Belief*, scientist and scholar Bruce Lipton tells us that the structure of our DNA changes as we open up to new ways of being and change ourselves by modifying how we look at the world. In our potential, source state, our DNA is tightly coiled, governed by the survival instinct and fear. Yet, when we discover the Divine potential within ourselves, a new structure emerges. Accepting our Divine state of being then fuels our climb to higher levels, where we become stronger, more aligned, and more joyful.

The second stage, or soul or "qi" level, is where we interact with the world. At this stage our efforts are focused on doing (outwardly expanding) or on being (focused inward). It is here that we can rewrite aspects of our inherited potential—actually improving upon our genetic design—by treating ourselves well and interacting positively with our environment. We aren't victims of our inherited DNA; we can choose our body's expression and experience. Ancient Chinese medicine refers to this principle as "tonifying our ancestors," meaning nourishing ourselves until the pool of our entire collective—past, present, and future—is improved by our own intention and attention to our own well-being. By embracing our Divine potential and living according to its dictates we can redefine our lives.

The third, or spirit, stage is where our Divine potential blossoms. This stage is where we completely uncoil to let our highest self emerge. We unclench and live to the fullest, free of all constraints. We open ourselves to the wonders of creation and unleash the powers of the universe to live our passion.

All of us have the ability to raise our energy from its primordial potential to its highest capacity and find the balance and happiness we seek. Using the vertical-horizontal energy grid to find balance within and without, you're going to learn to recognize and utilize all of your energies to break away from habits that have kept you stuck in unhealthy patterns, and to empower you to gain control of your body, mind, and spirit. As the Serbian proverb says, "Be humble, for you are made of earth. Be noble, for you are made of stars." You are made of the earth and stars. I encourage you to follow The Way to find your deepest purpose and express it joyfully—to learn what makes the earth move and the stars dance for you.

How I Transformed My Own Genetic Blueprint

My passion for my work is directly related to my personal experiences with the healing power I discovered in the Tao and in traditional Chinese medicine. I was born into circumstances that left me feeling alone and unworthy. As a teenager and then an adult I felt ill-equipped for life and had little confidence. Eventually, I spoke with a tremor in my voice and believed I was utterly worthless. I didn't know how worthwhile I was or even how worthwhile it was to be alive. I did not recognize the spark of the Divine inside me, only the story line I was living. Because of that my potential was not realized.

I tried to overcome my lack of self-worth by going overboard in trying to prove myself worthy. I chose partners I thought would make me feel better about myself, not those who were actually good for me and I for them. I smoked, drank too much, exercised too much, worked too much, and defined myself by how I looked and by what others thought of me. Of course, none of this helped—I still was unable to reach my highest capacity.

Not, that is, until I found the Divine spark that was tightly coiled within me. After years of reckless behavior, I found my way back to myself. When I lost all hope, I surrendered to life and found the place of stillness inside. And when I became still, I started appreciating the inherent joy of living. I realized that simply by being alive I was worthy.

With that understanding, I was able to move away from the purposeless and exhausting life I was living, in which I was constantly trying to prove myself, and toward using my talents to reach my highest good. I created new boundaries for myself. I chose healthy relationships. I learned to live from a place of joy rather than fear. My unhappy circumstances gave me rich fuel for my ultimate transformation and I grabbed that fuel and ignited it. Now I live following my own Divine guidance choice by choice, without stress (unless I choose it), moment by moment. In this way my life keeps getting better. The universe keeps providing, beyond my wildest dreams. I am so grateful that life gave me the opportunity to rise from the source level into which I had been born to higher, more joyful states of being.

2

Discovering Your Imbalances and Blocked Energy on Your Path to Creative Freedom

望 *Observe*

Like the moon, come out from behind the clouds.
Shine.

— THE BUDDHA

When you follow the teachings of the Tao, you live more observantly. You pay closer attention to the little things inside your universe, such as how deeply you are breathing. You also pay closer attention to things throughout nature—blossoms and ant colonies and the wonders of the night sky. By doing so you stay conscious that all of life is indeed miraculous and you begin to relate to it from a place of purity and wonder.

When you live according to the principles of Chinese medicine, you become more internally aware so you can more clearly see ways in which you might be stuck in unhealthy patterns of behavior. This recognition lets you shift the patterns into new, healthier ones that are in sync with your higher awareness.

Understanding Your Energy Sources

Anything that gets in the way of experiencing life in all its Divine aspects is considered by Chinese medicine practitioners to be an imbalance—and in many ways our society has become quite imbalanced. Instead of being attentive to the eternal, endless abundance that is within us, we are conditioned to pay attention to our aches and pains, to the news media, to negativity, to all the stressful actions that demand our immediate attention. This conditioning causes the mind to gradually close to the positive and the creative and forget the wonders of our universe. This has led to limited creative opportunity in schools and dwindling support for the arts. And being disconnected from the creative stream just leads back to further imbalance.

This chapter will give you tools to explore and identify whether any of the five expressions of energy are out of balance in your body. The following chapters focus on unblocking those energies, finding balance, and resuming living in a harmonious state.

Energy imbalances upset the mind-body-spirit complex and create stress, hormonal imbalances, fatigue, unhappiness, infertility, and internal discord, all of which cause "dis-ease." But practitioners of Eastern philosophy don't believe in fighting disease—disease is not considered an enemy. Instead, disease is overcome by raising energy vibrations to a level at which the disease can no longer manifest and falls away on its own.

This process begins by paying attention to symptoms of disharmony. Every little discomfort in your body, every disturbing thought, every so-called negative emotion is a knock at the door of your awareness that says, "Pay attention," which you must do. Unheeded warnings can become stronger and stronger. A bit of tension in the neck can lead to headaches, to an eventual stroke, even death.

In Western medicine, pathology is the study of diseased tissue. However, in its original Greek, pathology means the study of suffering—not being at ease with what is. Suffering, disease, and pathology are caused by resisting what is. When disease is perceived as an enemy, as something to resist and fight, it gains strength from the resistance. For example, taking an aspirin for a headache without discovering the headache's source enables its return because we didn't learn its cause; we simply addressed its symptom. When we view an imbalance through the lens of compassion and love, however, rather than as an enemy, we learn from its presence in our lives, accept its message, and allow the dis-ease process to dissolve.

Western medicine has a complex array of ammunition with which to treat disease. I feel lucky to have access to it when one of my children has a raging case of strep throat. But Western medicine doesn't keep us healthy—its focus is on treating disease rather than supporting wellness. In ancient China, doctors were paid only if their patients stayed well. Today, the "health" community is rewarded only when people become sick or diseased.

Eastern medicine works within the framework of what is to encourage the restoration of health. It meets us where we are, so that we can express the full potential of what we can become.

Uncovering Your Patterns of Living

According to the Tao, there are seven stages of life that take us from conception to death: primal essence, or pure potential; becoming; distinct being; having a sense of self; expressing oneself; living through acquired conditioning; and following ingrained patterns. Within each stage is an opportunity to move forward by paying attention to our body's messages and overcoming those things that are holding us back from reaching our highest destiny.

The following evaluation tools will help you look deep within yourself to uncover your patterns of living and learn how they differ from patterns in sync with your true nature. They will uncover the darkness within you so that you can begin to live from the light of your spirit.

The Yin-Yang Questionnaires

The following questionnaires will assess your balance of female and male qualities. As mentioned in the introduction, traditional Chinese medicine and the Taoists view all in terms of two opposing forces known as yin (–) and yang (+). Just as electricity requires opposing forces to flow, life requires opposing forces to create energy.

The yin and yang within us can become imbalanced. For example, if too much of our yang, or active side, is flowing too strongly, we can burn out—from our careers, our activities, our families—by not taking time for rest. On the other hand, if our yin, or more gentle side, is flowing too strongly, we may disengage from everything and do nothing but rest.

As you can see, the two polarities have extremely different characteristics, but yang is not better than yin and yin is not better than yang. Both are necessary; what is important is that they remain in a state of harmony.

Yang—Strong, Giving Tendencies	Yin—Gentle, Receiving Tendencies
Are prevalent in the upper part of the body—back, right, exterior parts of the body	Are prevalent in the inner part of the body—front, fleshy parts, left, inside of the body
Are prevalent in the stomach, intestines, gall bladder, urinary bladder, male sexual organs—that fill and empty	Are prevalent in the lungs, spleen, liver, heart, kidney, uterus, and ovaries—that hold specific functions
Cause us to be active, get things done	Cause us to be passive, allow life to happen
Are light, bright, vibrant	Are dark, shaded, hidden from view
Are external, superficial, focused on the outside and doing	Are interior, deep, focused on going within
Are dominated by the sympathetic nervous system	Are dominated by the parasympathetic nervous system
Are positive, moving forward	Are negative, allowing you to stay in the same place
Are dry, arid, used up	Are wet, moist, fertile
Are hot, hectic, restless, frenetic	Are cool and calm
Are loud	Are silent
Are busy, engaged	Are still
Are vigorous, lively, energetic	Are receptive

Our society, however, favors yang qualities over yin. Most rewards are given for action, not for looking within. It's acceptable to ask people who are being introspective, "Why aren't you doing something?" In other words, value isn't perceived in contemplation. But it is important to balance activity with rest. Turning external focus inward allows us to renew ourselves and prevents us from exhausting our resources. Seeds don't constantly produce. They gather strength within the dark, damp depths of the soil so they can burst forth with life. A fertile field must have fallow time or it won't produce a bountiful harvest.

Women are emotionally and physically more yin. The distinctly female pituitary hormones oxytocin and pitocin promote passive qualities and the ability to resolve conflict through bonding with other females. Long ago, women were valued for their fruitful, abundant natures and it was their very connection to nature, to the ebb and flow of life, and their ability to give life that conferred that value. But when our cultures started becoming more externally oriented, women were shamed and punished for their connection with the forces of nature. Author Joan Borysenko tells the story of when, as a little girl, she questioned the nonexistent role of women in the synagogue. She asked her rabbi the reason for this discrepancy, and he responded that women don't need a house of worship to be connected to the spirit of life; they inherently are connected. They bleed with the moon. They give life. They flow with the world through their emotions. Men, however, were seen as needing a house of worship because they connected with the spirit of life more from their thoughts and their intellect.

This story reminds us that along with women, men's yin qualities have also been stifled, so that men, too, are not able to embrace their softer tendencies. Yin, in every form, has declined. Women have become much less focused on who we are inside and taught to focus attention on how we appear to the outside world. In an attempt to create more balance, women now strive to be more like men, developing their musculature, sucking in their bellies, and rejecting aspects of their femininity, such as being open and receptive. In my own case, because I perceived my parents were dissatisfied having yet another girl in the family, I reacted to this perception by acting like a boy. I kept my hair short, played sports, climbed trees, and tried to be tough. When I grew up, I retained the male attitude of doing and achieving and kept strengthening my exterior to cover up the softness inside. I starved myself and exercised like a maniac to make the curves disappear—I literally made myself infertile.

We each have an inner yin aspect—trusting, intuitive, open, and flowing—and we each have an inner yang aspect—direct, confident, authoritative, and goal-oriented. By identifying your yin and yang tendencies using the exercise below, you will become aware of your imbalances and grow from that understanding. For example, if your yang is too strong you may be relying too much on your intellect, while not letting your feelings impact your decisions. You may be prone to rigidity and imposing your will on others. If your yin is too strong, you may be extremely sensitive and emotional and lack an inner voice, losing yourself to others. Understanding your imbalances is the first step toward bringing your yin and yang back into alignment.

Yin exploration

Write down your first response to the questions that follow, and contemplate how these answers have shaped your life:

1. When you were growing up, how did you feel about being a girl?
2. What kind of messages did you receive about the value of being female?
3. How did you feel when you had your first period? Where were you? Who was with you? What did you do?
4. Which of your feminine attributes gave you a sense of pride or self-worth as a child?
5. How did you know your mother loved you? How did she show her love?
6. How did you show your love to your mother?
7. Who were your female role models?

Yang exploration

1. How did you know your father loved you? How did he show his love?
2. How did you show your love to your father?
3. Who have been the important men in your life? What did you learn from each of them about masculinity?
4. How do you think your life might be different if you were a man?
5. How old were you when you first had intercourse? How did you feel about it?
6. How do you feel about intercourse now?
7. How do you experience arousal?
8. What do you do with that feeling?
9. If you are in an intimate partnership, how is your relationship with your partner?
10. How do you show affection to your partner?
11. How does your partner show affection to you?

Yin-yang exploration

1. Identify and make a list of your feminine and masculine qualities. Feminine examples could be receptive, fertile, internally oriented. Masculine examples could be active, powerful, goal-oriented.
2. Which of these qualities work for you and support your cherished destiny? Which do not?
3. In which situations do you act more from your feminine nature? In which do you act more from your masculine nature?
4. When do you feel out of balance?
5. When do you feel in balance?
6. What can you do to bring more balance into your life?
7. Your endocrine and reproductive systems consist of both masculine and feminine aspects. So do your attitudes about your reproductive system. Which masculine or feminine traits do you attribute to your feelings about your own fertility, your inner creativity, and your sense of sexual arousal?

Now that imbalanced responses have been brought into the light of your conscious awareness, when you notice that these imbalances are showing up in your behavior, you can allow their resolution through intending a more balanced response.

The Five Energy Tendencies

Energy tendencies are metaphors for aspects of nature that repeat themselves over and over again: earth, metal, water, wood, and fire. These tendencies show up in our personalities, emotions, interactions, and bodies. They create our energy field: the way we think, feel, and relate to ourselves and others. When our energy field is strong, nothing can penetrate it; negative messages from magazines, the Internet, television, billboards, news, and nonsupportive coworkers and family members cannot get in.

Earth energies

Drawing the energy of the earth to the center of the body, represented by the spleen and the digestive system, creates a strong earth energy field. To assess how well your earth energies are functioning, consider how well you are maintaining boundaries in your life. Are you pulled in too many directions at once? Can you say no when you need to?

Metal energies

Metal energy signifies contracting and expanding tendencies, the ability to come together and release. The lungs are the organs that carry this energy. To assess how well your lung energies are functioning, consider how much in life you are willing to release or let go. Are you clutching onto any person, thing, or situation that causes you to feel tense? Can you envision its release? Can you remember times in the past when it felt wonderful to let something go?

Water energies

Water energies always seek to go deeper, and search for crevices to seep into. Water energies are represented by the kidneys, and to assess their state you need to determine how much you can love yourself—even love the dark shadows within yourself and the way you express your authentic self in the world. Even the shadows are made up of the same spirit source as the rest of all of creation. Are you courageous enough to look at what you're really made of? Will you go into the depths and embrace what you find?

Wood energies

The wood element refers to the force contained within a tiny seed that enables it to develop into a sequoia. In our bodies, this energy is represented by the liver and is powerful and free flowing. To find out the state of your own liver energies, ask yourself how free you feel in your life right now. What situations make you feel trapped? What makes you feel free? Can you discern which aspects you need to accept and which you can change?

Fire energies

The fire energies are hot and expansive and are represented by the heart's circulation, which has an outward movement. To assess the quality of your fire energies, ask yourself how much love you can extend to the world. Can you forgive what you don't like? Can you envision yourself loving everything? Can you see the possibility of opening up just to love and finding that everything is perfect?

Discovering Your Character Tendencies

Each element defines certain characteristics of the human personality. You may find that you align almost entirely with one type of energy. If you do, you need to watch to ensure that its tendencies don't become excessive. On the other hand, you may find that you don't gravitate at all to one particular element, which means you may lack that energy and need to apply more effort to wielding its power. In either case, don't be alarmed. Many people have ample tendencies in one to three categories, but are lacking in one or more—very few are balanced throughout the elements and they need to build up or reduce one or two. I, for example, have the most water and earth tendencies, am strong in metal, and almost lacking in wood. Thus, I have to watch for and address the sluggish tendencies of earth, water's propensity for isolation, and a weakness in wood's tendency to exert itself in situations that call for more strength.

As you go through the elements, become aware of how these tendencies can predispose you to react in certain ways, helping you to accept yourself as you are and to live in a more fulfilling way, in harmony with all of life.

Character tendencies

Earth people are centered, stable, and naturally nurturing of others. These strong earth mothers are the shoulders we all go to to cry on. They are warm and love to give affection. They value and tend to their homes, inviting friends to the warmth of their hearth. They tend to have a few good friends to whom they are fiercely loyal. Earth people value stability, harmony, and sustenance and can make a banquet out of a shoe. Yet they can become overly stable and sluggish. They also have difficulty making decisions that take them out of their comfort zone. Because they are natural caretakers, they often lose their own boundaries and can have difficulty with self-care. They naturally worry about those they love and like as well as those who aren't close to them. Earth people can benefit from a hobby in which they can totally lose themselves, removed from obsessive concerns. It is helpful for earth people to vary their routine, rearrange their house, and do something for themselves every day.

Metal personalities value appearance and order. These detail-oriented people are disciplined and self-controlled, organized, meticulous, and discriminating. They value beauty and art and tend to be fastidious in their appearance as well as the aesthetics of their surroundings. They are natural analysts and accountants and can be counted on to care for priceless assets. They tend to see themselves as righteous and enjoy sanctified rituals. Those with imbalanced metal tendencies, however, have difficulty with disorder and spontaneity. They may become critical of others and have difficulty living with chaos and expressing emotions. They may wear a façade of clenched control and loathe the day when their order is upset. People with metal imbalances can have difficulty loosening up. Because they aren't naturally impulsive, it can be helpful for them to pretend to be silly until the freedom feels good. Wearing one thing that doesn't match the other things they're wearing can get them used to the spontaneity of life.

Water tendencies are drawn toward the depths, and often like dark colors like navy blue and black. Water people value intelligence, wisdom, and insight highly. They tend to be quiet, with almost a moaning quality to their voice. They are insightful and enjoy philosophical discussions and reading. They are perceptive and ingenious, and value being and knowing more than doing. Water people are honest, but they aren't as comfortable as their sisters in social settings. Sometimes it seems as if they view life hiding behind a bush, evaluating the safety and purity of a situation. They are independent loners, preferring to go with the flow, and may appear a bit guarded. They aren't prone to give affection easily, and yet can be pierced to their core. They value depth in others. They also have acute, sensitive hearing and, while they tend to sleep well, ambient sounds can keep them awake at night. Water people tend to be on the lookout for the perfect teacher in life. However, imbalanced water tendencies can make these people prone to withdrawing from others and becoming isolated. Risking contact with others, though, and allowing themselves to be vulnerable can pull them back into balance.

Wood people usually have strong, forceful personalities. They know what they want and can get it. Drawn to the color green, wood people can express their confidence and assertiveness, enjoy making things happen, and can easily bring their imaginative dreams to reality. Wood people have a great inner vision and are seers. They aren't easily hindered by boundaries, but are movers and shakers who take charge and become powerful leaders. Their ability to initiate action and run their plans decisively allows them to get things done. However, their intensity makes them prone to frustration when the world doesn't participate in their plans. They often have difficulty falling asleep at night and can be prone to high blood pressure. Sometimes wood people find it difficult to relax, and tend to collapse rather than ease into rest when they do. Too much wood can make one feel invincible, separated from the rest of the world. Wood people need to work at remaining flexible and taking time for relaxation daily so that they can recognize their own limits and find peace within.

Fire personalities are joyful, lively, and communicative. They embody the fiery red tendencies that ignite excitement around them. Always open to the next opportunity, they bring with them passion and delight. They might be a bit talkative, the natural life of any party, and they long to unite with others and receive admiration. Fire people are charismatic communicators and can make friends with anyone they meet. These natural lovers tend to be expressive and affectionate, but might be a bit clingy, not recognizing where they end and another begins. Their strengths are not in deep contemplation and preparing for the future; they tend to live in and embrace the moment. Because they are drawn to intimacy and unity, they tend to have difficulty going within and conserving their energy for tomorrow. It is helpful for fire personalities to walk quietly by themselves every day and recognize their strength in solitude.

Rebalancing your tendencies

As so many people do, as a child and a young adult, I denied my true nature. Though I didn't understand it at the time, I was strong in water energies, in gathering and looking within, but I longed to be popular and vibrant, like the girls who were strong in fire energies. After a few drinks, I found that I could be like those girls, and alcohol became my tool for becoming what I perceived to be more valued by society. But while alcohol took away my inhibitions and made me socially acceptable in my own eyes, it eventually became my downfall, because it made me act in a way that wasn't me. When I finally became still again and looked deeply within myself, I was able to understand that if I continued to live according to an outer authority, I would utterly lose myself. Eventually, I began to accept my solitary nature and even learned to honor it. I started to live authentically, happily, as the person I truly am.

Fiona, a beautiful British woman who attended a Fertile Soul retreat, married when she was forty-two years old. She had been a successful professional analyst but gave up her career soon after she married. When she arrived at the retreat, I found that emotionally she felt purposeless; physically, she had relatively severe allergies, asthma, and respiratory ailments. When she filled out the character tendency analysis she gauged herself as almost all metal, with no earth tendencies at all. So I suggested that she explore some creative ways to discover her inherent earth energies, which would help her to find passion as well as love herself and others.

After she left the retreat, she dreamt about a garden where she felt peaceful and happy. Although she had no experience with gardening, she created a small garden in her backyard and found that she enjoyed spending time there, connecting with the earth. Little by little she expanded her garden, and found more and more pleasure placing her hands deep within the earth and making new life grow. As her peonies and rosebushes blossomed, Fiona felt a renewed sense of passion and started nourishing herself as she fertilized and nourished her garden. Her respiratory allergies completely resolved.

As you go through the rest of the chapters, be aware of how your own tendencies impact you on every level—physically, mentally, emotionally, and spiritually. For example, if you found that you lack water energies, it's likely you'll find that you have a problem with, or an imbalance in, your kidneys. Now, that doesn't mean that you will have kidney problems your entire life, but you may develop a propensity for kidney difficulties if you don't work at keeping them healthy. The body is so incredibly adaptive that organ systems borrow energy from one another to maintain balance as much as possible. Every symptom is a call for help.

Once you become aware of your imbalances, the ten secrets to wellness will show you how to correct them, eliminate blockages, and lavish your body, mind, and spirit with loving attention and care to live a healthier, more fulfilling, more blissful life.

The Seven Stages of Life

According to Chinese medicine, our original energy, or essence, unfolds according to an evolutionary blueprint that is initially governed by prenatal influences and later by influences of the life process. The seven stages of living are landmark periods that signify how we make choices based on the ego self that take us away from our true nature. As you read, remember that each later stage contains opportunities for awareness and for finding your way back to the Tao, and that it is never too late to live a fertile life.

Stage I

The first stage of life is the fetal stage. When our parents' yin and yang are magnetically attracted, their egg and sperm fuse to produce the blueprint for a new human being. This primal essence draws the soul into human form and imprints it with a unique nature willed by heaven. As long as the fetus remains within the womb, she has no sense of individuation and remains pure potential, like a seed, yet is influenced by the mother's response to her environment during gestation. The womb is the portal between the void and this plane of existence.

Stage II

The second stage of life begins as the infant accepts her first breath. It is thought of as the stage of "spontaneous self-becoming." The infant is connected to all of life, but still has no sense of individuation. Like a bud, she comes into this existence as pure potential, sparked with a unique expression of divinity, her soul, which is meant to unfold throughout the rest of her life. During this stage she is subconsciously conditioned deeply by the environment in which she is growing up.

Stage III

The third stage of life is childhood. The child becomes conscious of herself as she learns her name and all about herself. She learns she is a separate identity distinct from her parents and siblings and finds myriad opportunities to become even more distinct and separate.

During this stage the child moves from the self-expressive spontaneity of childhood into more external awareness. Watch a young child dance, uninhibited and unself-conscious, still a pure expression of being. When she starts to dance for others, she loses her spontaneity and begins to forget her original face as she develops her own self-image. Deep wounds can occur at this impressionable phase of identity, especially if her image becomes tainted by messages of negativity and shame.

Stage IV

During this stage, the teenage years, yin and yang divide and set the stage for the loss of original nature. As teenagers learn more about the world, they lose touch with their true nature and begin to define themselves according to others. "I have the power to create: I have hips. I like black. I am cool. I like tall boys. I am mysterious. I like horses. I see myself as fat so you must see me as fat, too." It is during this stage that she begins to reject heaven's will and assert her individual will onto the world. But the ego has an agenda ("I must be skinnier and cooler in order to be happy") and that becomes a theme that colors her response to the world. My theme during these years was, "I can never be good enough."

Wounds can contract us into acting out negative life themes at this stage. For example, Janice grew up being sexually abused by her older brother, someone she had loved and respected. When the abuse worsened into rectal penetration, she became deeply ashamed and left home. Rather than enjoying the self-defining phase of adolescence, she lived the pathology of metal and became rigid and withdrawn.

She also developed the most severe case of painful endometriosis I had ever seen, in which her bowel became enveloped by the lining of her uterus. When Janice ovulated, her rectum, instead of her uterus, produced copious amounts of mucus, and each period brought on severe menstrual cramps and rectal bleeding.

After being involved in a deep spiritual quest that took her out of her body, Janice came to the Fertile Soul retreat. Although she had been able to remove herself from the pain her body was experiencing, she hadn't found a cure for her mental and emotional pain. After spending time with her, I determined that I needed to bring her back into her body in order for her to heal emotionally. But it was incredibly difficult. As I performed acupuncture on her, it was hard to keep her in the treatment—she closed her eyes to escape. But after a month of doing qi gong (pronounced "chee kung"), Chinese breathing exercises, she learned to remain in her body, even during pain.

When Janice came to a second Fertile Soul retreat, she stayed in her body during further acupuncture treatment, and that was when our souls connected. I can't tell you where I placed the needles; I just know I was guided to where they needed to go. As I placed them, a shift occurred and the energy of the room changed. Janice lunged on the treatment table and gasped in fear as her entire body undulated with a great thrusting force. But from then on, her monthly blood flowed from her uterus and her pain lessened. By accepting her body and no longer resisting what was, the cellular memories that Janice had embodied were released. She now lives happily, healthfully, and passionately, studying the ancient Incan cultures in Machu Picchu.

Stage V

Throughout Stage V, the young adult filters everything she sees and does according to the self-defining patterns established in the preceding stages. As a young adult I lived through the filter of needing to prove that I was good enough—I defined myself by my relationships, what I was doing, and how I appeared to others, a way of life completely reinforced by Western society.

Fortunately, it's always possible to ignite the light of awareness within and learn to recognize imbalance. Rose was a top young movie producer in New York City, but her stress-filled career had begun to take its toll on her health. While she was fiery by nature and thrived in her adrenaline-rich profession, her constant need for external recognition deprived her of a true sense of self and resulted in an intestinal malabsorption syndrome. Concerned for her health and well-being, Rose left her high-powered job and began acting out children's stories in a New York City school district. By nurturing herself and letting go of the need to define herself by her profession, she became able to express her creative force and helped others learn to express themselves. As she adjusted her lifestyle, her digestive system regained its health as well.

Stage VI

As an older adult, if she hasn't yet been shocked into awareness, her false sense of self may become more deeply ingrained. She becomes a creature of habit and reinforces her unhealthy posturing by getting a new car, a new profession, a "boob job" or facelift, a new boyfriend, or a new family. But no one has to remain stuck in this damaging way of life. Anyone can break away from conditioning and return to her original nature.

The husband of a friend of mine had an affair when he turned fifty. My friend, in turn, got breast implants and dyed her hair platinum. Now, when she looks back, she realizes how immature both her own approach and her husband's were to dealing with the inner voices that told them they needed to find themselves. Once they listened and looked at themselves, they found that their external changes did not bring them what they needed. By finally becoming aware that they were not living the life they were meant to live, they began a journey of more fruitful self-discovery through couple's therapy.

Stage VII

If she has been conditioned to push past resistance and has not listened to the warning signs in earlier stages, her negative patterning may now be her physical undoing—she may experience high blood pressure, alcoholism, heart attacks, and strokes. But even in Stage VII, it is not too late. She can still wake up to her habitual negative patterns of self-expression and take the pathway home to her original nature.

It is never too late. With every breath we take and with every beat of our heart, we can connect to the call of the Tao and come back to ourselves. Jean, a retired municipal judge, spent most of her reproductive years on oral contraceptives. She married later in life to a man with grown children. Jean had strong wood tendencies and felt as though she imposed herself on the world without looking inside for sustenance. In her early sixties, she contracted breast cancer and had bilateral mastectomies; she felt that part of the cause of her cancer was that her reproductive and creative energies had been squelched her entire life.

After spending time at a retreat and following the ten secrets, Jean was able to let go of her rigidity. She began to appreciate the gift of life and rediscovered her connection to the ways of nature. She began posing in the nude for art photographers and at age sixty-five learned to belly dance, eventually teaching belly-dancing classes. She felt as though she were growing younger rather than older and had a complete physical, mental, and spiritual rebirth. Jean's "golden years" became golden indeed.

No matter which stage you are in or what type of life you are leading, you have unlimited opportunities to transform yourself. Your story line has brought you to where you are now, but it does not need to continue to define you. At the Fertile Soul retreats, women tell their stories the first day. Then they learn to expand beyond the limitations of their stories and let them go. You have already begun to shine the light of awareness within your temple—now it is time to rebuild it. The rest of this book will show you how to take down restricting walls, open the blinds, rearrange the furniture, and develop a new plan for living—in the palace where you were always meant to be.

Through the course of nature,
Muddy water becomes clear.
Through the unfolding of life,
Man reaches perfection.
Through sustained activity,
That supreme rest is naturally found.
Those who have Tao want nothing else.
Though seemingly empty,
They are ever full.
Though seemingly old,
They are beyond the reach of birth and death.

—Tao Te Ching

Part II
The Ten
Ancient Chinese
Secrets to Relieve
Stress, Renew
Energy, and
Fulfill Your Most
Cherished Destiny

Secret 1:
Balance Your Energies—Physical, Emotional, and Spiritual

和 *Harmony*

Our cup is the full moon; our wine is the sun.

— IBN AL-FARID

Women are not machines; we are attuned to the rhythms of nature and act in accordance with its laws. As the philosopher Chuang Tzu wrote in the second century BC: "Heaven, Earth, and I are one, and all things and I form an inseparable unity." We are linked to nature through an invisible web joining cause and effect, substance with substance, and energy with energy. As we abide by the laws of the universe, we tap into and

37

unleash incredible powers of healing and creativity. We create our life as we would have it be.

Balancing energy is at the root of all traditional Chinese medicine and wellness practices. As you read in the previous chapter, you are actually energy—the same energy that burns in the sun and flows in the ocean. Initially, I couldn't fathom the concept myself. In fact, when I first studied traditional Chinese medicine I argued with one of my professors about the interchangeable nature of energy and matter. According to my Western medical training, a cell was a cell, lab values were lab values, and the human body was an ever-deteriorating disease process just waiting to exhibit a symptom so medicine could intervene. When I challenged my Chinese teacher, she humbly told me, "Perhaps you should just listen, or you could look up Einstein's theory of relativity in the library." So I forced my ears to listen and my mind to open to the myriad possibilities it had been closed off to during my Western upbringing and my Western medical training.

In order to practice Chinese medicine effectively, I had to continue to open my mind beyond the confines of what I had been taught. Originally, learning about the body's limitations made me view the body and life itself as somehow deficient. Now I started to examine what my patients' life responses were showing me. As I treated women as the miracles they are, their incredible responses shifted what I was looking for. When I looked for disease, I found it. When I focused on wellness, healthy patterns revealed themselves. As those who came to me for help improved, this wisdom caused a new thought pattern to emerge within my own life. I learned to pay attention to what life is, and has always been, trying to teach me—that what I focus on is what I create in my life.

The Universal Energy Force

By opening my ears and my mind, I learned that human cells and tissues conduct and transfer energy through molecules throughout our bodies, giving us life. The Chinese call this universal energy force qi, which is described this way in the classic Chinese medical text, the *Neijing*:

> *The root of the way of life, of birth and change is Qi; the myriad things of heaven and earth all obey this law. Thus Qi in the periphery envelops heaven and earth, Qi in the interior activates them. The source where from the sun, moon and stars derive their light, the thunder, rain, wind and cloud their being, the four seasons and the myriad things their birth, growth, gathering and storing: all this is brought about by Qi. Man's possession of life is completely dependent upon this Qi . . .*
>
> *Let's open our eyes to the mysterious wonder of energy.*
> *The root of the way of life, of birth and change is Qi . . .*

In the human body, qi manifests in several different ways. First, it is a kind of bioelectrical force that is carried throughout the body by an extensive network of channels called *meridians*. These channels, which are formed from the remnants of embryonic folds, are invisible to the naked eye yet have been mapped over thousands of years through observation and experimentation by Oriental physicians and can be felt when you attune yourself to the subtleties found in the background of life. Applying pressure or attention at different points along the meridians produces *measurable, demonstrable effects* on different body parts, organs, and systems.

Second, qi is converted in the body into fluids and the vital substances yin, yang, and blood that make the body run. Each fluid and substance works within the different organ systems to carry energy throughout the body and to help convert what we take in—air, water, and food—into the nourishment our bodies need. Then these fluids and substances transport the nourishment to our organs, cells, and systems and later remove them from our bodies.

Third, qi is part of our different organs and systems. This means that specific acupuncture points can be used to treat specific organs. For instance, heart qi moves through a channel that runs into the chest, down the inside of the arms, and to the little fingertip. Directing intention, acupressure, needles, magnets, or even your own breath to these positions will affect the flow of qi through the meridian and, in turn, affect the functioning of the heart and spirit, which it controls. While energy cannot be seen or heard, its effects determine our health or disease. If energy is blocked it cannot flow, and if it cannot flow, function is compromised and disease results, on the physical, emotional, or spiritual plane.

When I first began my work with fertility, my initial goal was to help women resolve their obstructed qi to help them conceive a child. After working with thousands of women over the years, however, I realized that not only had previously infertile women become fertile, but their physical and emotional blockages had been resolved as well. Their lives were changing and getting better. They were moving their homes, pursuing new careers, having new ideas, even releasing spouses who weren't supporting their highest good. They were clearly expressing their creative energy in many ways and no longer settling for anything less than they deserved.

Helena developed ovarian cysts when she and her husband, Thad, were trying to conceive their second child. Her body was giving her a sign, and she learned to listen to it. She discovered unhealthy patterns in her marriage, and she subconsciously thought that if they had a son, her husband would be more supportive to Helena and attentive to their four-year-old daughter, Megan. When Helena and Thad began working to resolve unhealthy patterns in the family, Helena learned that Thad didn't want another child, as he felt financially pressed to support Helena and Megan. They decided a son would not fix anything, and as they developed better communication and support skills, the family of three thrived, and Helena's ovarian cysts went away. The following year Helena and Thad adopted a younger cousin's unwanted son.

When energy is allowed to flow smoothly, it is possible to create good health as well as well-being. Even emotions like anger can be blocked or free-flowing. When appropriately expressed, anger actually improves our response to negative events, like certain cancers. Anger released in an appropriate setting is healthy and necessary. Free-flowing energy strengthens muscle, detoxifies the liver, and clears the skin. If energy is obstructed, however, the growth process can give rise to tumors or cancers— all illness arises from going against our creative nature. When blood flow is obstructed, for example, a condition called blood stasis results, making the body prone to varicosities, fibroid tumors, and potentially deadly blood clots. When emotions such as anger are blocked, a person's face gets red, the blood can feel like it's boiling, and blood vessels in the eyes become red and congested; over time, habitually holding in anger may cause

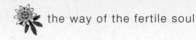

migraine headaches, high blood pressure, and strokes. When stasis is resolved, however, it results in an emotional condition the Greeks called ecstasy. We need to unblock stagnating energy wherever we find it to restore the body's natural balance and live at a more healthful and stress-free level.

Restoring balance to qi

In Chapter 1, I talked about the body's horizontal and vertical energy grids and represented the five energetic tendencies in the shape of a cross, represented below by a four petaled flower. To refresh your memory, the base of the cross, the source or "essence" level, represented by water, is our physical, deepest, most dense level. The arms of the cross, represented by wood, earth, and metal, the soul or "qi" level, represent how we carry

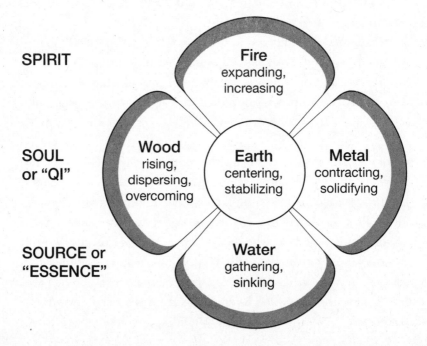

out the beliefs of our mind and emotions as we interact with the world. The top of the cross, the spirit level, represented by fire, signifies the highest state of being. Peace and joy come by balancing the physical self with the soul and the spirit.

The cross can also show how each of the five energy tendencies has a corresponding physical, mental, emotional, and spiritual component.

❋ **The gathering, sinking energies**—These energies represent our basic survival instincts. In order to maximize and balance these source energies, ask yourself these questions:

1. How often do I allow myself time to be alone? (Be certain to allow some time alone every day.)
2. How often do I meditate or allow my mind to relax with a hobby or pleasurable project?
3. How do I feel about myself, irrespective of my job, friends, partnerships, or status in life? (Evaluate how you feel weekly.)
4. Do I love myself first?

❋ **Rising, dispersing energies**—These energies represent our ability to overcome resistance to things that keep us stuck in bad patterns. To maximize and balance these soul energies, ask yourself these questions:

1. Which areas of my life am I tolerating simply because it takes too much effort to change them?
2. Which areas of my life keep me stuck?
3. Which areas can I change?

❋ **Centering, stabilizing energies**—These energies govern what we allow into our lives. To maximize and balance them, ask:

1. Which innate qualities define me?
2. Who or what supports or doesn't support these qualities?
3. Is there any action I need to take?

❀ **Solidifying, compacting energies**—These energies bind us to people, places, things, and situations and give us a sense of order and control. To maximize and balance them, ask:

1. Which partnerships define me? (Ideally, very few.)
2. Which people, places, things, or situations do I need to release?
3. What masks of self identity am I ready to relinquish?

❀ **Expanding, increasing energies**—These energies, usually hidden by obstructions in other tendencies, are innate expressions of the inherent hope, love, and joy of life. To maximize and balance these spirit energies, ask yourself:

1. Which activities allow me to completely lose myself or lose track of time?
2. How do I express the unadulterated joy of being?
3. Who can I love without needing anything in return?

Balancing energy in the body

Now we're going to look at the grid in yet another way to learn how energy obstructions can negatively affect organ systems. These exercises will help you evaluate whether energy systems are functioning smoothly and optimally. For example, if your libido is strong but you experience hot flashes, you likely are deficient in kidney yin. Or you may have excess heat from another source.

However, for now we are only evaluating imbalances, not interpreting what they mean. There are no right or wrong answers. The questions are meant to raise your level of awareness about each of the energetic systems.

If your answers indicate imbalance, the following chapters will give you the keys for opening up obstructed energies.

Organ function is governed by the five energy elements. The **source level**, represented by water and the kidney system, governs

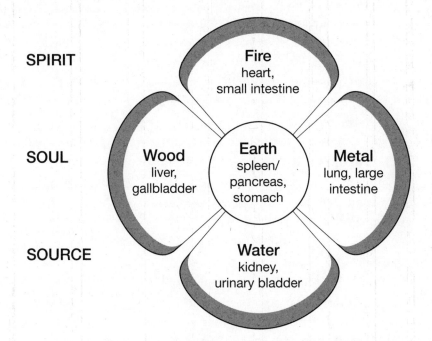

our sexual energies, our hormonal output, and our water elimination. To discover blocked kidney energies, ask yourself these questions:

1. How well do I eliminate fluid?
2. Do I have difficulty holding my urine, do I urinate too frequently (more than seven times per day), or does the need to urinate wake me from sleep?
3. Is my libido strong enough for me?
4. Am I experiencing hot flashes and night sweats?
5. Do I experience pain or weakness in my structural foundation (my low back or knees)?

The **soul level** is represented by wood, earth, and metal. Wood governs the liver system, which oversees our ability to overcome internal stress. To discover blocked liver energies, ask yourself:

1. How well does my body process new changes?
2. Do I tend to hold onto physical ailments a long time?
3. Does it seem that some areas inside my body just aren't functioning smoothly?
4. How can I move more pleasurably?
5. Are my tendons and joints stiff?
6. Do I feel like my body needs to decongest and detoxify?

The **earth** aspect of the **soul level** is also represented by the spleen, which governs digestion, absorption, and blood production. To uncover blocked spleen energies, ask yourself:

1. How is my digestion?
2. How many times do I chew before I swallow?
3. Do I feel adequately nourished?
4. Do I take nutritional supplements?
5. How well do my muscles move?
6. Do I practice movement every day?

The **metal** aspect of the **soul level** is also represented by the lungs, which govern how well we're protected from and separated from the outside environment. They govern elimination and release of old cells and worn-out relationships and patterns as well. To uncover blocked lung energies, ask yourself:

1. How deeply do I breathe? Does my belly expand when I inhale or does the breath remain up in my chest?
2. What or whom do I have difficulty letting go of?
3. Do I exfoliate, sauna, or brush my skin?
4. Do I have a bowel movement every day?
5. Do I take in enough fiber?

The **spirit level** is represented by the heart, which signifies the highest self that wants to share and express itself in the world. To discover blocked heart energies, ask:

1. Do I feel anxious and impatient?

2. Does my heart beat rapidly or erratically during times of stress?
3. Can I allow myself time to simply relax and be?

Balancing the emotions

Now look again at the grid to understand how energy obstructions can negatively affect emotions.

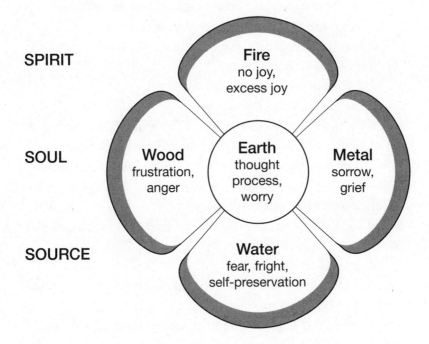

To see which energy level—source, soul, or spirit—is being blocked and causing you the most difficulty, consider these questions.

❀ Source—Kidney energies

1. Am I afraid that I, alone, am not enough?
2. Am I worthy of having been created?

❀ Soul—Liver energies
 1. Am I easily frustrated?
 2. Am I prone to anger, resentment, or rage?

❀ Soul—Spleen energies
 1. Do I feel as though my mind can't stop churning?
 2. Do I worry a lot?

❀ Soul—Lung energies
 1. Do I feel lingering sorrow about things in my past?
 2. Are there past losses that I can't seem to overcome?
 3. Is it hard to release and move on?

❀ Spirit—Heart energies
 1. Whom or what do I love fully?
 2. Do I experience joy in my life?
 3. Can I look at a flower, smell fresh air, and feel the immensity of creation, or is it hard for me to forget myself?
 4. Do I sometimes feel the need for excessive excitement?

Balancing spiritual energies

Now look at the grid to understand how energy obstructions can negatively affect the spiritual self.

❀ Source—Kidney energies
 1. Do I feel as though I have a destiny or a higher purpose?
 2. How do I honor it?
 3. How do I acknowledge my innate self, the reason I was born?

❀ Soul—Liver energies
 1. How active is my imagination?
 2. Do I dream and follow my intuition?
 3. Do I have goals and aspirations?
 4. Do I feel as though I am more than just my physical body?

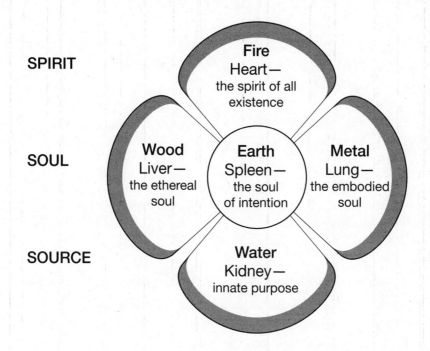

SPIRIT

SOUL

SOURCE

Fire
Heart—
the spirit of all
existence

Wood
Liver—
the ethereal
soul

Earth
Spleen—
the soul
of intention

Metal
Lung—
the embodied
soul

Water
Kidney—
innate purpose

❀ Soul—Spleen energies

1. Can I envision using my power of intention to create my life exactly the way I want it to be, rather than letting my thoughts control my life?

2. Can I allow myself to focus and concentrate on what is right in front of me?

3. Can I look at a sunset without being distracted by thinking about anything else?

4. Do I eat mindfully, paying attention to what I bring into my body?

5. Do I live mindfully, paying attention to what I bring into my sphere of being?

❀ Soul—Lung energies
1. How connected do I feel to the rest of the world?
2. Can I share my core self with others without binding myself to them?
3. How many unhealthy relationships can I let go of?
4. How do I surrender control of the outcome of things?
5. Have I ever experienced the state of raw abandon?

❀ Spirit—Heart energies
1. Can I dance with joy by myself?
2. Can I love someone without requiring that the person love me in return?
3. Can I appreciate the inherent joy of living life fully?

At this point, you have begun to recognize how energy is flowing in your life. Some energies may be balanced, and you may be content in these areas; other areas may have revealed obstructed energy patterns. In certain areas you may have discovered significant blockages that seem difficult or impossible to rectify. Paradoxically, that is where the healing begins. Self-awareness initiates the process of transformation.

The energy has a directional component because it's contracted in your physical body, so it manifests in the organs, emotions, and energies of the soul, as shown by the cross of flower petals that groups them all together on the next page.

In the following chapters I'm going to expand on what I've talked about here with information on lifestyle changes, and meditation exercises that will help you unblock and enhance the imbalanced tendencies you've recognized so that they flow robustly and unobstructed throughout your body, mind, and spirit.

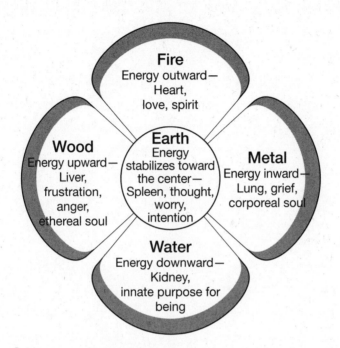

This is the miracle of life:
that each person who heeds himself
knows what no scientist can ever know:
who he is.

—SØREN KIERKEGAARD

Secret 2: *Let Yourself Be Who You Are*

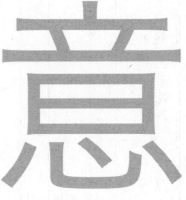

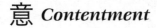 意 *Contentment*

Instead of trying to be a mountain,
Be the valley of the universe,
So all things will come to you.

— Lao Tzu

A great deal of emotional and physical imbalance comes from resisting your natural self. Many women spend their lives striving to become like the women society holds up as ideal. The media inundates us with pictures of wafer-thin models with tiny hips, tinier waists, and large breast implants, and gives us the message that we are not enough as we are, that no one is perfect. This modern vision has evolved from the creative pleasure of the fashion industry and those who follow it. In its continuous search for the new look, the dominant aesthetic has strayed further and further from women's natural beauty. Women are soft and curvy, valleys ready to receive, strong in their connection to life. Struggling toward an unreachable ideal results in stress and pain.

Contentment begins when you accept your deepest, innermost self, when you allow your natural self to be. As you find happiness in the present, you allow even more happiness to come through. Chinese philosophy holds that water, the universal source element, gives you the innate potential to create—art, ideas, houses, technology advances, happiness, books, tools, babies—and live contentedly.

Water is the mother of the universe, the very wellspring of existence. Just look at water's myriad manifestations: a droplet of mist, a bubbling brook, a fresh, clean rain, a rushing river, a waterfall, a deep ocean, a glacier, morning dew. It is water's nature to receive and unite, to separate and to bond in an unbreakable force. Water, like no other element, changes its shape and always goes deeper, eroding even the hardest of surfaces.

In the body, the kidneys govern water. The *Neijing*, the classic Chinese medical text, tells us: "The kidneys are responsible for the creation of powers. Skill and ability stem from them." The kidneys represent the potency of the life force and the foundation of the body's yin and yang.

Cultivating Inner Peace

According to Chinese legend, the Original Vessel created the universe. From the swirling cosmic bliss of primal chaos, the Original Vessel experienced the urge to become. This caused a shattering—a division of everything light from everything dark. From that shattering, heaven and earth were created and divided. The light rose and the dark sank, resulting in tension between the two opposites.

The Original Vessel sacrificed herself to become all that is. The old dissolved into the new, producing polarities, or opposite forces, that in turn produced friction. Wholeness shattered and transformed into distinct and separate parts.

That is the initial story of creation. Yet after being separated into distinct manifestations of possibility, the parts must be reintegrated to enable the creative process to continue and to prevent complete chaos. As creation evolves into a higher state of being, higher order is constantly reestablished. However, as we move toward that higher level, some chaos remains. The Taoist process of alchemy asks us to courageously shine the light of awareness on our inner chaos, and accept its presence so it can be transformed into wisdom. With practice, it's possible to focus on your true inner voice and transcend perceived limitations and painful memories because you view them authentically and without fear.

Our source, or kidney, energies help us to move to that higher level of being. It is the seed of potential

The kidneys are represented as a tight spiral of potential that merges with the soul and the spirit. Like a morning glory that emerges each dawn from a tight spiral to a five-pointed blossom, so does our true spirit expand and become joyful, carried on the current of our bubbling source energies.

The Three Levels of Water Energies

The water energies express themselves at three different levels. It's possible to determine if your water energies are imbalanced and the simple exercises I provide can help to bring them back into alignment.

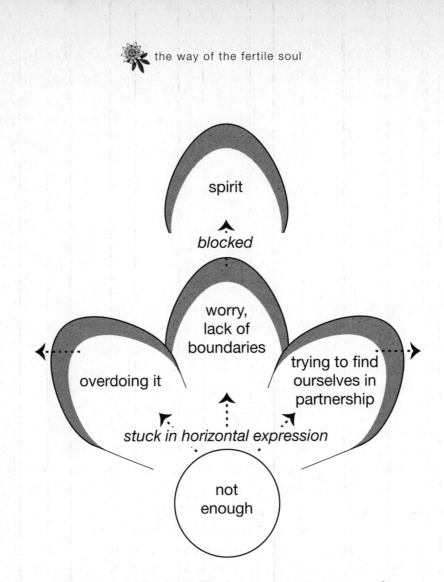

The lowest level—believing you are not enough

The lowest level of the source energies is the part you hide from others. This level contains the sludge at the bottom of your being, the leftover chaos that tells you, "I am not enough. I am inadequate, and need to prove myself." But this foul sludge is the fuel for transformation. By finding and facing it you can draw strength from it and begin to live your purpose.

I lived most of my life at this first level of source energies. I felt unworthy and constantly needed to prove myself. But one day I hit a breaking point and I could no longer run from myself. When I was forced into my own depths, my empty vessel became filled from the bubbling spring within, and a prayer that I had heard many years before rose into my mind: "Relieve me of the bondage of self." That prayer set off a current of power within me and I suddenly needed to run. I recited the prayer out loud to myself as I ran into the bathroom. I curled up in a fetal position on the bathroom floor. Exhausted, I went to the depths of my darkness. There I found stillness. I heard a voice from deep inside that was louder than the voices of my parents and friends and partners that I had allowed to drown out my self.

That inner voice told me simply, "You are worthy." But that message changed my life. My foundation restructured itself. A sense of peace swept over me and changed the way I looked at everything. I realized that I was worthy—because I lived and breathed I had worth, something I hadn't known until that horrible, despairing, preciously magnificent moment.

The second level—living authentically

Marjorie's midlife had been so focused on being a wife and mother that her entire sense of self was tied into the well-being of her husband and two sons. Within two very trying years, her boys left home, her husband divorced her, and he left her feeling utterly alone with no clue about who she was or what she was capable of doing with her life. Marjorie was brought to her knees in despair, as her life as she knew it was over. At age forty-nine, she found a job as a school secretary and got an apartment; as her depression passed, she found herself drawn to music. As a girl, she had been a rather proficient pianist, but

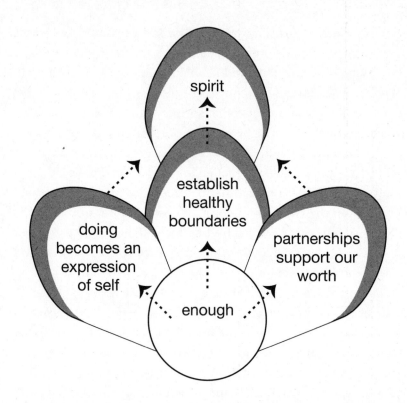

was told she couldn't make a living playing piano. She allowed herself to sing, and when she could afford it, she enrolled in guitar lessons. She now makes her living as a singer, motivating other women to find their inner passion.

The second level of being emerges from the acceptance of the truth that you are enough. At the second level you live abundantly. Everything you do reflects your inner being. At this level you live your purpose, whether it is digging ditches or writing beautiful music—whatever you do, you do with a strong sense of self and with all of your creativity and strength. At this level you understand that you can no longer do anything that compromises your true nature. You can't stay with a partner or employer who doesn't treat you with respect. You support your innermost self with a sense of sufficiency and acceptance. As Mary Oliver says in her poem "The Journey":

> . . . *and there was a new voice*
> *which you slowly*
> *recognized as your own, that*
> *kept you company*
> *as you strode deeper and deeper*
> *into the world,*
> *determined to do / the only thing you could do—*
> *determined to save / the only life you could save.*

The highest level—expressing abundance

Influential women throughout history like Pocahontas, Joan of Arc, Susan B. Anthony, Anaïs Nin, Florence Nightingale, Helen Keller, and Indira Gandhi possessed an innate strength that gave them power to change their world and those around them. We all have it, but not all of us know we possess this power.

At the third level you overflow with your own power. You become a fountain of unlimited strength, like a geyser. Your true inner self connects to your spirit and you become aligned with the highest energies of the universe. At the third level you are constantly fulfilled and joyful. Because you nurture the root of your being, here you remain well and exhibit the highest state of being—physically, mentally, emotionally, and spiritually.

Discovering Your Water Energy Imbalances

Who we are depends upon the deepest aspect of our kidney energies, our life's purpose and destiny. When waters are calm, they reflect deep inner harmony. Imbalanced kidney energies

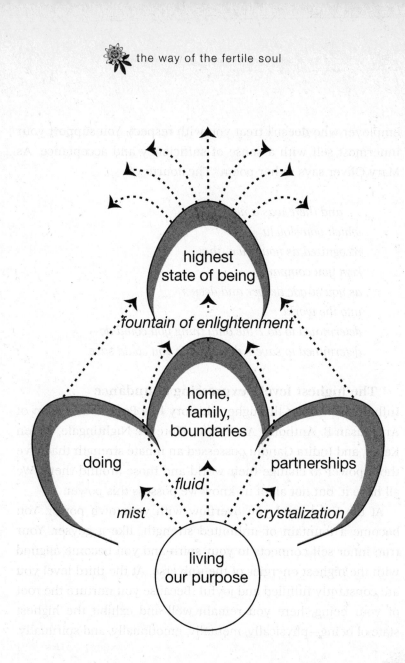

may express themselves as lack of self-love, purpose, or sexual energy. Physical manifestations of a general kidney imbalance include weakness, soreness, and pain in the lower back and knees, where the kidney channel runs. People with waning kidney energies will often have dark circles under or around their eyes. Kidney weakness may be further differentiated into kidney yin deficiency, which might be accompanied by signs of vaginal dryness, dry eyes, premature gray hair, dizziness, ringing in the ears, hot flashes, and night sweats; while lacking yang energies might result in symptoms such as low libido, profuse vaginal discharge, frequent, dilute urination, urgent, early-morning loose stools, dull, cold-menstrual cramps, frigid extremities, and feeling cold most of the time.

If you suspect that you have these imbalances, it doesn't mean you need to rush out to see a doctor; you need to care for your foundation, your kidneys, by facing fears and looking within. Water energies should be replenished daily to keep the inner wellspring flowing. Choose to not wear yourself out by running on stress hormones, but become quiet, like a still pond, and take respite from the world.

Strengthening Your Water Energies

If you've determined that your water energies need support, the following exercises will help you to appreciate them, connect with them, and unleash their power. In addition, eating foods such as pumpkin seeds and alfalfa sprouts (seeds and sprouts have immense energy potential and feed our foundation) supports the essence of the kidneys, as do B vitamin supplements and colloidal minerals. If your hormones are at a low ebb, indicated by an irregular menstrual cycle or a low sex drive, Chinese herbal tonics can help. If you aren't familiar or comfortable with herbal remedies, find a good naturopath to help point you to quality products. Be sure to check with someone knowledgeable before adding therapeutic herbs to an existing medical or natural treatment, to protect against unwanted interactions.

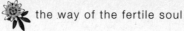

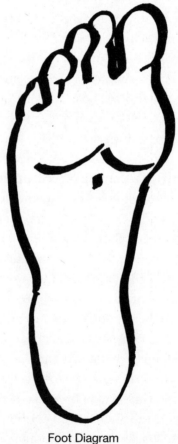 Meditation: Becoming grounded

This exercise helps strengthen you at your foundation: your feet. The meridians (channels where energy flows) that lead to the kidneys begin on the bottom of each foot, located between the center and ball of your feet. While you are sitting or standing, you may bring intensity to your kidney energies by feeling the bubbling spring that is their source, and drawing it up into your body, as roots draw up water from the earth.

Foot Diagram

Pay attention to the subtle but firm force that connects you to Mother Earth. Once you feel the energy, bring that feeling up into your legs, sacrum (the base of the spine that joins to the hip bones), and spine. Feel the warm, bubbling water energy nourish your bones.

To nourish yourself further, care for your feet—not by having pedicures but by making them feel good. Walk barefoot more often. When you walk on grass, sink your toes into the soil and feel your connection to the ground. Before you go to bed at night, soak your feet in Epsom salts. Treat your feet well so that they can carry the weight of the day.

Meditation: Connecting to the source

Many of us are energetically top-heavy, focusing most of our attention above the neck. This exercise will help make you aware of your major life source, the Dan Tien, or "chamber of essence," in the lower abdomen. It will shift your attention inside your body, and give you a sense of strength from deep within.

Root yourself to the center of the earth by being aware of the bubbling spring point at the bottom of your feet. Next, concentrate on the area a few inches below your navel, called the chamber of essence, where your uterus resides. Your most powerful energy, or qi, resides in this sea of energy deep within your center.

Feel yourself breathing in and out through your chamber of essence. Let your belly button lead your breathing and fill up your lower abdomen with the qi of life. With your mouth closed, place the tip of your tongue behind your upper front teeth and breathe up your midline. Bring your attention to the area between your vagina and anus. Tighten the perineal muscles

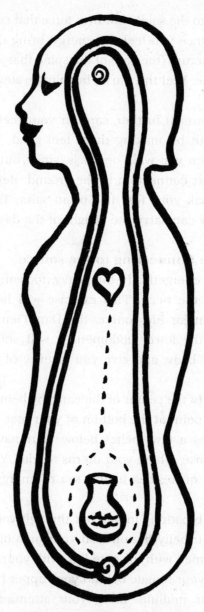

Chamber of Essence Diagram

there and pull energy up from the vaginal canal into and through the reproductive organs. Bring your focus to the life source, the uterus, and continue to breathe in, letting your breath pool as your lower abdomen expands. Inhale, up past your belly button, past your heart, and up to the area between your eyebrows. At the end of the inhalation, lift the energy to the top of your head. As you exhale, allow your qi to shower down along your neck and spine to the tip of your tailbone. With the next inhalation, scoop your sacrum up toward the perineum and repeat the circuit. (Note: Some women find it easier to reverse this flow, breathing down the front and up the back.)

Continue to breathe into your pelvis, expanding and contracting your lower abdomen with every breath and filling the pelvic bowl with fresh, clear qi. Moving your energy along this microcosmic orbit will enliven you with the power of the universe. This series of attentive movements is most effective when practiced daily. Try the exercise now and plan some other times to try it. Eventually it will become a natural part of your self-care rituals.

Meditation: Counting your blessings

Taoists believe that the spine and brain are extensions of the kidney energies and that the spine must be supple and fluid to support healthy organ functions. To strengthen the spine, and therefore the kidney energies, do the following exercise.

Beginning at the tailbone, mentally count your vertebrae, visualizing each bone and nurturing it with your attention. The bones represent your core self. Next, bring your attention to your sacrum, which houses your sacred sexual energies and is the root of your psychophysical structure (the word sacrum means "sacred place" in Latin). At the bottom of the sacrum is a hole

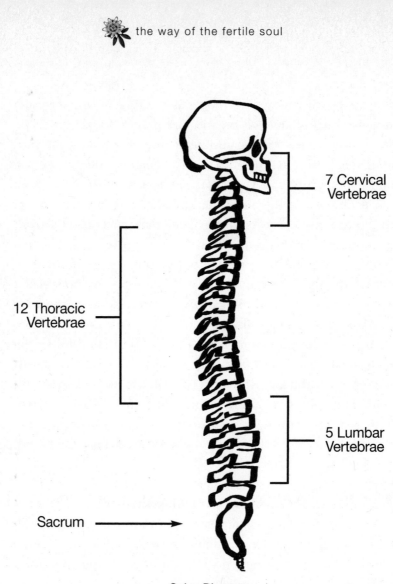

7 Cervical
Vertebrae

12 Thoracic
Vertebrae

5 Lumbar
Vertebrae

Sacrum ⟶

Spine Diagram

through which massive amounts of energy pass. Feel this energy pulsing into the bottom of the sacrum and feel your sacrum moving back and forth as you breathe, as if it, too, is breathing.

Now shift your awareness to the five lower lumbar vertebrae, paying attention to their immense support. Then greet and feel

66

each of the twelve thoracic vertebrae onto which your ribs attach to encase your heart and lungs. Next, connect with your seven cervical vertebrae, which run up your neck to the base of your skull. Then, pay attention to the back of your head, your temples, and your face bones. Finally, think of the top of your head as an outlet for the bubbling spring that is moving through your body. Let yourself become a fountain of energy that begins at your feet and emerges through your head. Feel the love it brings and appreciate the body, mind, and spirit it nourishes. Smile internally with tenderness and with all of your being.

Meditation: The womb breath

This exercise is particularly useful in helping let go of fear. There is nothing wrong with being afraid; you just don't want to let fear control you. Fear causes the self to withdraw and stay continually on the alert for protection. The remedy is to acknowledge the fear and breathe into it, to go quietly to the dark, scary place, feel your fear, watch it, acknowledge it, see it for what it is, and then release it by breathing it out through your nose. By pulling your energy downward, to the source, the chambers of essence, and then drawing it up to your highest state of being, you accept your fear and gently allow it to dissolve.

Focus your breath a few inches below your belly button, as if you are breathing in and out through the chamber of essence. As you breathe in, picture your depths as a deep, dark blue, the color of water, which governs the kidneys. Picture your uterus, a pear-shaped organ with fallopian tubes extending from the top, as a void that connects you to all of the cosmos, a void into which the power of the universe is allowed. Locate your uterus and massage it. Then bring your awareness to your ovaries,

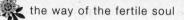

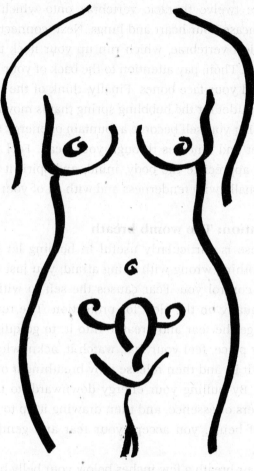

Organ Diagram

which lie between your hips and pubic bones, deep within, and massage them as well. Let your reproductive organs know that you care for them, enlivening their creative function. Breathe into them.

As you breathe out, feel your kidneys in your lower back, on the left and right sides of your spine, just beneath your lower ribs. In stillness, appreciate the energies of your kidneys. Connect with their wisdom and let go of the stress that overworks your adrenal glands.

Yolanda found the courage—which comes from the French word *coeur*, or heart—to face her fear. When she came to her first Fertile Soul retreat she was forty-eight, and had spent most of the previous five years trying to conceive after marrying a man eight years younger. She arrived at our diagnostic session full of apprehension. Spreading out her medical charts in front of me, she asked with anguish, "Is it too late?" After going deeper with her, I said, "Yes, it is too late for you to conceive naturally." I knew that wasn't what she wanted to hear, but it was the only hope for her transformation.

Although tears spilled over as she realized her fear had become reality, eventually Yolanda was able to relinquish the empty hope within and accept the truth. By being courageous she was also able to see that though her theme in life had been to provide her husband with a child, because she thought he needed one to complete their future together, she had never really wanted a child herself. Her courage also enabled her to recall a dream from her childhood: to help orphaned children throughout the world. Once Yolanda found and accepted her true nature and reality, she was able to live her dream, and now works with orphans. She found and applied the courage to create a new world.

Being yourself

Allowing yourself to live according to your true inner nature enables you to immerse yourself in life, to love, to express compassion, to create, and to accept things the way they are, which opens you more readily to improvement. In many ancient languages, there is no word for "artist" because it was recognized that we are all creators. Take a minute now to remember your first creative experience—was it drawing a picture, planting a seed, singing a song? Now think about what you are creating in your life right now—what are you making manifest? What something are you making from nothing? What options are you opening up? What energy are you expressing? Are your creative acts sacred to you? Are they enlivening your spirit? Do they express your deepest self? Are they supporting your highest good? Ask yourself these questions each time you start an endeavor, and become still so that the inner voice that answers is louder than the outer voices that surround you. By listening to that inner voice you will live an abundant life and be your own true fountain of plenty.

> Can you focus qi into such softness
> You're a newborn again?
> Can you be female, opening and closing heaven's gate?
> Give birth and nurture . . . without possessing.

—LAO TZU

Secret 3:
Find and Embrace Your Inner Spaciousness

敞 *Openness*

To the mind that is still,
The whole universe surrenders.

— LAO TZU

When women truly accept themselves for who they are, and feel fully comfortable within their own skin, they open up to something bigger—a sense of wonder and possibility. However, many people take on more than they can comfortably handle, trying to fill feelings of lack, the shameful worry that they're not good enough. But keeping excessively busy with stressful jobs, relationships, and routines only adds to bad feelings, stress, and exhaustion, often causing health to suffer. Many women ignore their bodies' messages until life forces them, through pain or illness, to really take care of themselves.

In everyday life this may mean letting go of an activity, a relationship, or a job. Internally this may mean turning our attention within to release tension that is held inside, realigning with our higher nature by focusing on our own health and well-being while we let the external world care for itself. By acknowledging the patterns that have served us in the past and allowing those that no longer serve us to dissolve, we enable our internal energy to flow, smoothly and unobstructed, bringing us to a state of true freedom. This inner spaciousness is essential to our well-being. Just as the emptiness of a bowl allows it to be filled, in this inner nothingness we find everything. When we're too busy—full of work, worries, responsibilities, guilt, shame—there's no room. Inner peace is necessary in order to have the inner reserves to power our own inner transformations—hormonal, emotional, or those that fulfill our visions and dreams.

The Wood Energies

The immense energies that drive internal transformations are referred to as wood energies—like the energies pushing a sprout through its seed casing to become an ash, a maple, or a pine that reaches up and out. In the body, the wood energies are represented by the liver.

The liver resides in the upper right-hand side of your abdominal cavity, tucked under your ribs. It is a large organ with many branches that reach out to purify the body of its toxins. The liver stores, filters, and regulates the blood supply, produces proteins, metabolizes hormones, and rids the blood of anything that is not useful. The liver represents new beginnings, just as the wood energies symbolize rebirth and move us away from thought patterns and emotions that keep us stuck in time. Liver or wood energies grow, expand, and generate.

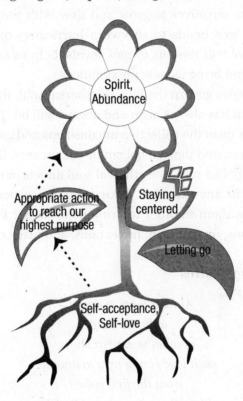

Think of the tremendous amount of energy required for an infant to become a teenager. That incredibly expansive energy is within you right now, governed by wood and depicted by the color green, the color of growth in nature. Your wood energy can take the power of water, which I talked about in Secret 2, and turn it into something new, the way water feeds a seedling and enables it to turn into a tree.

The wood energies take us from where we are now to our future. But they can be very uncomfortable: resisting the change may cause pain, leading us to try anything, such as taking anti-depressants, to make the pain go away.

If we allow ourselves to grow and flow with the world—the way a palm tree bends to survive a hurricane—our powerful wood energies will raise us to new levels, help us survive passing storms, and bring us new possibilities.

Wood energies govern the *hun*, or ethereal soul, that aspect of all people that has always been and always will be. The ethereal soul connects us to the collective unconscious and governs intuition, aspiration, and the symbolism of our dreams. Described as rarified energy like mist, the ethereal soul directs our movement through life in any direction, taking our life experiences and learning from them in order to bring us to higher levels where creative visions, imagination, projections, and plans can arise.

Fulfilling desires

Always there is desire—
only the shape
of what is desired shifts,
each love giving way to another
from the first sound
of heartbeat inconceivably there.

— JANE HIRSHFIELD

In addition to moving us forward, the wood energies also promote aspiration. While many spiritual traditions have difficulty with external longing, traditional Chinese medicine teaches that the creative power of yearning can manifest in happiness and fulfilled dreams. The greatest obstruction to healthy liver function is living in a state of unfulfilled desires.

The Taoist way is to reduce desires, not attempt to fulfill them. Taoist philosophy teaches that when we wish for something, we must not hold on to its outcome. Dreams and hopes may become intent that leads into action, but it's important to let go of the outcome. Holding on to what we think should happen produces suffering; unfulfilled desires can result in anger and resistance. For example, here's the way some women try to fulfill their desire to have a baby.

She desires a child. She tries to conceive. It doesn't work. She tries harder. It still doesn't work. She prays that God will bring her the child she desires so deeply. She may even bargain with God to make this happen. She goes to see a doctor. The doctor says there is something wrong, but can try to make her pregnant through this or that intervention. She tries it. It doesn't work. She tries harder. She prays harder. It still doesn't happen. She gets frustrated, angry, depressed, and further and further away from her goal.

This is a typical reaction to a desire that someone fears may not be fulfilled. Children often use this approach—a forceful yang approach that goes only toward the light, rather than dealing with the dark, or the yin aspect of the situation. This approach only recognizes the desire, not what it takes to manifest the desire. But taking care of the depths can help to transform our lives and reach a higher level of fulfillment.

In contrast to the ego-driven approach, look at how the creative Taoist works to fulfill the desire to have a baby. She desires a child. She tries to conceive. It doesn't work. *This is all this approach has in common with the previous approach. Instead of trying the same thing over and over again, expecting a different result and becoming more and more frustrated when it doesn't*

75

happen, a follower of The Way lets go, allowing creation to occur. When someone surrenders this is how they view desires:

She stops struggling. She looks at what needs to be adjusted in her world in order to allow her desire to manifests. She says, "I align myself with the creative force of the universe, so that creation—be it a new relationship, a new profession, a better state of health, a new interest or purpose, or a baby—may come to be. I look at the contrast in my life that is preventing growth and creation and I release it."

Wood energy imbalances

Wood energies give us the strength to overcome obstacles, just as trees have the power to break out of a seed casing, imbed in the ground, drink in moisture, emerge through the soil, become a seedling, then a sprout, then a shoot, and then weather the vicissitudes of nature to grow strong and tall. Wood or liver energies also allow us to leave harmful situations and empower us to say no when that's what we need to say. The liver imbues us with the power of anger, so that we can overcome resistance. But the liver also regulates the smooth flow of emotions. Healthy liver energies allow us to feel frustration, express anger, and then release it and let go of any outcome. These powerful, regenerative forces allow us to both overcome obstacles and accept what comes.

Liver energies that are unhealthy or imbalanced, however, depleted through blood loss, an overactive life style, too much stress or exercise, or too little rest and self-care, lose their ability to smooth the emotions. Then even small annoyances can become exaggerated and result in frustration, and we become inflamed with anger that results in self-hatred, depression, or rage. If these conditions persist, the liver loses its ability to transform and it becomes difficult to glide through life.

Overwork, in particular, can result in disturbances of the liver. Many workaholics resort to the escape valve of alcohol to overcome internal tension caused by overwork, which worsens the effect on the liver. When wood energies become disturbed, women may try to force their way into the world and resent others for not playing according to their rules. They may get stuck in the unfulfilling horizontal plane of mere survival and feel increasing internal pressure and an inability to relax.

Overdoing, drinking alcohol, and resisting your natural inclinations create obvious imbalance, which blocks you from your true center. Manifestations of liver imbalances include migraine headaches, vision difficulties, light sensitivity, heartburn, high blood pressure, premenstrual tension, abdominal bloating, and breast pain. Difficulty falling asleep at night due to inner frustration indicates stagnated liver energies as well, as does having a bitter taste in your mouth—literally and figuratively.

Inner stillness or inner spaciousness nourishes a healthy liver. So when you feel your blood pressure rising and there is no appropriate action to take, retreating to your inner stillness to meditate on your source can help you regain your strength. Life is a fluctuating interplay of action and withdrawal. If it is time to draw back but you continue to act, your soul will send you messages that you need to retreat. Those messages may come in the form of tension between the eyes, conflict with coworkers, or infertility, and if they don't resolve through physical or emotion-based solutions, life may provide a boost by taking away a job or a relationship that is hindering your highest good.

Finding Balance

Karen was an excellent example of a body out of balance. While she appeared to be in good health, her periods stopped in her mid-thirties and her doctor found that she had premature ovarian failure and was in menopause.

Instead of listening to the messages her body was sending her—that something was wrong—Karen tried everything she could to force a period. Her doctor put her on prometrium and it didn't work. Instead it caused an increase in the level of prolactin, a hormone that causes lactation at the expense of ovulation: attacking the first symptom had only caused another symptom to occur. So Karen's body, in its infinite wisdom, had simply shut down the entire process.

When Karen's issue wasn't corrected by her reproductive doctor's treatments, she turned to me. I discovered that she had liver qi stagnation, the Chinese terminology for unresolved inner stress. When I discussed my finding with Karen, I told her that I could resolve the immediate physical manifestation of the stagnation, but I couldn't prevent it from returning. She would have to discover what was causing the problem.

Karen later revealed that her husband had lost his job and become very depressed. The couple was strapped financially, and Karen couldn't stand her husband's attitude about their situation. The two rarely made love, and Karen had begun to work more and be at home less. Her husband stayed home and watched television, and when Karen was home she made dinner, cleaned the house, and became ever less fertile. Not long after we talked, Karen's husband went out of town for several weeks of training and during that time Karen ovulated and menstruated. Once her husband returned home, her periods stopped once again.

Now, it doesn't take a brilliant diagnostician to determine what was behind Karen's lack of periods. Perhaps her body was showing her that bringing a child into the family at that time would only magnify the couple's problems, and it was protecting her from conceiving. Other mammals don't go into heat when their environment is overly stressful.

Karen's initial attitude impacted her ability to recognize the truth of her situation:

- ❀ I was meant to have a child.
- ❀ I've always wanted a child.
- ❀ I finally found the perfect man and he lost his job.
- ❀ I'm starting to believe my doctor's opinion that I'm too old to have a baby. (Note that the doctor's attitude is not a fact.)
- ❀ My period won't ever come.
- ❀ I am not ready to have a baby with a donor egg and my doctor says that's my only option.
- ❀ I don't like my life, and my husband doesn't like his life.
- ❀ I nag my husband constantly and still nothing gets done.
- ❀ I am turning into my mother.

Despite her attitude, Karen needed to recognize and accept the facts of her present situation:

- ❀ I want to have a child.
- ❀ I haven't had my period in six months.
- ❀ My husband lost his job just over six months ago.
- ❀ Prometrium didn't work for me.
- ❀ When my husband was gone, my period came.

Then she needed to identify her feelings about the facts:

- ❀ I am scared I'm too old to have a baby.
- ❀ I feel hopeless.
- ❀ I'm afraid my husband and I will get divorced and I'll end up alone.
- ❀ I'm afraid I will never have a child.

Next, she had to determine what she could not change, and therefore needed to accept in order to relieve her stress:

- ❀ My age
- ❀ My husband's attitudes, behaviors, or job status (she could have divorced and remarried but chose not to)
- ❀ My doctor's opinions about my reproductive status
- ❀ The outcome of whether my period will come
- ❀ The outcome of whether I will become a biological mother
- ❀ I am not my mother

She also had to determine what she could change to relieve her stress:

- ❀ My response to my husband
- ❀ My attitudes about my health and reproductive status
- ❀ My diet, eating plan, nutritional supplements
- ❀ My exercise regimen, meditation schedule, activities

Once she understood all of these factors, Karen developed a plan for what she needed to do:

- ❀ I will work eight hours per day—no more.
- ❀ I will tell my husband how his behavior makes me feel. I will ask him to make dinner for me when I work all day.
- ❀ If I come home and the house is messy, I will hire a housekeeper.
- ❀ I will tell my husband what I will and will not allow, and let his actions be his own.
- ❀ I will do qi gong breathing exercises every morning for fifteen minutes.
- ❀ I will do an emotion meditation exercise every evening before bed.

Karen also learned how to recognize symptoms of impending stress: When I try to control my husband's behavior, I notice a tightening beneath my diaphragm. My breath gets shallow. Then she determined how she would respond to those symptoms to prevent stress:

❀ When I recognize this tightening, I relax, breathe deeply, and consciously release the tension.

❀ I identify the feeling in my abdomen, which I usually feel as anxiety and frustration.

❀ I tell my husband about it if he is available to me. Otherwise I call my sister or a friend.

As it turned out, Karen was not too old. A woman's age is often used to discount other life issues. As she and her husband incorporated an empowered attitude toward improving their life situation, his training turned into a new job, Karen managed her home life, her hormones and periods returned to normal, and they eventually became parents.

Eight steps to receptivity

Whatever the reason, if you're not vibrantly healthy and happy, this is merely a symptom of an underlying imbalance. To find the imbalance and resolve the problem, look deep inside and think about your life as Karen did. Then answer the eight questions that helped Karen, to discover your own path to accepting yourself and your situation.

1. What are my attitudes?
2. What are the facts?
3. What are my feelings about the facts?
4. What can I not change and therefore must accept?
5. What can I change?

6. What is my action plan? (Be specific.)

7. What are my symptoms? (To uncover deeper symptoms, bring your attention to your right midsection. Connect with your powerful liver energies. Ask yourself, What do I need to rid myself of? What do I need to overcome? Where are my energies resisting life? Let your awareness circulate within.)

8. How do I respond to my symptoms? (See below for techniques for resolving the symptoms.)

Embracing your inner spaciousness

Releasing inner conflict frees up energy that can be used to transform and create new possibilities in our lives. To resolve wood imbalances, connect with the power of your imagination. See yourself expressing health and abundance and having your dreams become reality. Turn your compassion to your inner body and appreciate the many functions of your liver. Feel a sense of reverence and gratitude. Breathe healing breaths into your liver. Meditate as often as possible.

Self-massage can also help bring your awareness to the tension in your body and help you resolve it and let it go. Massage your feet, your temples, and your belly with a mint-based oil, which helps release obstructed energy. Massage your breasts to lift stagnated liver energies there and prevent further buildup.

For people in generally good health, I also suggest trying an occasional liver cleanser, involving fasting, detox teas, and avoiding toxins by switching to organic foods and by staying away from toxic fumes and cleaning supplies. Look online or check with a naturopath or other practitioner of natural medicine for some good liver cleansers.

Also pay attention to your body's reactions to your world. Work on accepting the things that you can't change and be courageous in working to change those things that you can. You'll find wisdom in that awareness, and you'll also find balance. The powerful "Serenity Prayer," written by Reinhold Niebuhr, helps me to determine where to place my energies when I become upset:

> *God grant me the serenity to accept the things I cannot change,*
> *Courage to change the things I can,*
> *And the wisdom to know the difference.*

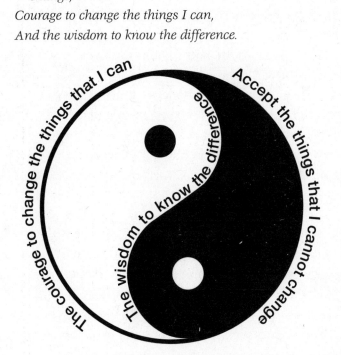

The journey to finding balance requires us to let go of the patterns that obstruct or cut off the flow of our life force. Another technique for recognizing both the patterns and the life force helps us unclench ourselves to enable an unobstructed energy flow. Are you clenched or unclenched? Become aware of the difference and check yourself routinely to remain fluid and free.

Clenched

To understand what being clenched feels like, make a tight fist. Press your teeth together and tense your jaw. Look around and compare yourself to others. See how different they are from you and how they have it better than you. Take small, shallow breaths as you recognize that they are younger and have flatter stomachs; suck your stomach in tighter. Turn your thoughts to all you don't have but desire and all the insurmountable obstacles in front of you. Think about all you haven't done at your job and your sense of hopelessness. Should you stay later at the office tomorrow or work through lunch? Become aware of the worry and stress you feel and think about how it will keep you awake tonight.

Notice the stress that these clenching attitudes produce. Can you feel how it creates contracting tension inside your body? Can you feel how stress and worry close off your energy and inner spaciousness?

Unclenched

To understand the sensation of being unclenched, start by releasing your fists. Open your hands and let your shoulders drop. Close your eyes and turn your attention within as you exhale. Breathe deeply, feeling the depths of your breaths as you let out your belly. If you're quiet enough, you may be able to hear the amazing sound of your heart beating—part of the miracle that you are.

Breathe slowly and deeply and let the knot of tension untie itself. Let your muscles relax, and think of something that makes you laugh. Notice the vibrations of your laughter and see if you can feel it reverberate throughout your body. Connect with the deepest part of your belly. Feel a sense of compassion and allow a smile to emerge. Feel for any residual tension anywhere in your body that is asking for your attention. Bring your awareness and the healing energy of your own hands to it.

Unclenching and allowing your energy to flow make all the things you do require less effort, which means you will expend less energy because you'll be functioning on a much higher level. When you unclench, you breathe deeper, your sympathetic nervous system relaxes, and blood flows to oxygenate your entire body. You actually increase energy and balance your hormones. Your digestive system can also absorb nutrients better and your intestines can properly excrete waste. Relaxation and pleasure chemicals are released in your brain and gut and you rest more deeply and can become more effective.

> *If you want to become whole,*
> *let yourself be partial.*
> *If you want to become straight,*
> *let yourself be crooked.*
> *If you want to become full,*
> *let yourself be empty.*
> *If you want to be reborn,*
> *let yourself die.*
> *If you want to be given everything,*
> *give everything up.*
>
> —Tao Te Ching

Secret 4:
Allow Life to Live Through You

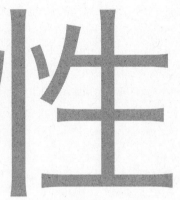

性 *Nature's Way*

When we lose our essential harmony with creation and exhibit a state of imbalance, where does the error lie? With Heaven or with man?

— HUANG DI (the Yellow Emperor, in the *Neijing*)

Heaven in me is Virtue. Earth in me is qi.

— QI BO (the Yellow Emperor's physician)

Life flows through the body's center by way of the solar plexus, which is located midway between the belly button and the bottom of the sternum. Here many nerves come together, digestive processes are controlled, and emotions meet. Our center is also a psychic gathering place where we create and reinforce our self-image. Deeper than the self-image, however, is a sense of self that isn't touched by our interpretations of life. This sanctuary, deep within our depths, was in our infant awareness before our thought process formed, and we can access this clarity by calming the reactive mind and allowing new inspirations to emerge. Habitual negative thought patterns sometimes block this clarity and blind us to our highest potential. One of my favorite examples of this is an anecdote about Albert Einstein. After years of intense calculations, Einstein's theory of relativity came to him while he was relaxing in the bathtub. He had to stop thinking about it before it could emerge.

The Earth Energies

The center consists of the spleen, the stomach, and the pancreas. But the spleen is the pivot around which the mind, body, and spirit rotate. Very importantly, the spleen is in charge of turning the food we eat into qi, blood, and other forms of usable energy and sending nutrients to the other organs, tissues, and cells. Spleen energy manifests in the gastrointestinal system and is markedly affected by what we eat.

The center governs what gets absorbed and what gets expelled by the body, separating the pure from the impure, the healthy from the unhealthy. It tells us when the food we eat isn't good for us and it also tells us when our thoughts are damaging our well-being. In traditional Chinese medicine, thought is governed by the same energies that govern taking in food and releasing its by-products. Just as our bodies become what we eat, our lives reflect what we think. Thoughts that follow negative patterns—such as feeling inadequate—lead to depression, stress, and hopelessness, and ultimately damage health. Reinforcing a negative self-image prevents the self from expanding its image and telling a new story. Pain in the gut, ulcers, or an irritable bowel are symptoms that may develop when someone spends more time listening to negative voices inside her head and out in the world than listening to what her gut is saying. When our thoughts support our highest mental and emotional functioning, our lifestyle and dietary choices tend to support our greatest physical health.

Beverly came to see me after her doctor told her that her thirty-six-year-old body was acting like that of a fifty-year-old woman. She later said it felt like he kicked her in the stomach. In other words, she internalized that message within her center. It reflected back in her beliefs, and she literally became like an old woman—her hair thinned and turned gray and her skin became wrinkly within a month of her doctor's devastating pronouncement. Working with Beverly, I helped her reprogram the message of decline by suggesting that she magnify her youthful properties and focus on her juicy qualities, like the way her body moved. Her body became younger by the day once she started listening to the messages of her own center.

Physical manifestations of imbalanced spleen or earth energies often show up in the digestive system. To discover whether your body is giving you signs that your earth energies are out of balance, ask yourself the following: Do you have a poor appetite or feel bloated after eating? Do you experience abdominal pain or loose stools? Do you crave sweets or tend toward low blood sugar? If you are fatigued, have low energy or low blood pressure, are prone to feeling heavy or sluggish, don't exercise, or have been diagnosed with hypothyroidism, look to your spleen system. If you bruise easily, have varicose veins or other bleeding problems, including thin, watery, profuse, or pinkish menstrual blood, also look to your spleen system. Weak musculature, excess (whole body) sweating without exertion, organ prolapse, hemorrhoids, polyps, diverticula, and poor circulation also indicate that the spleen energies need to be nourished.

Spleen energy is called earth energy because, just as the earth draws energy through its core, we draw energy from our core, or spleen. Like the earth, the spleen can become too dry or overly wet, and then, like the earth, cannot properly nourish those that rely on it. When it is too dry from lack of fresh, whole, nourishing foods, the spleen can no longer absorb necessary water, which leaves the body quickly in the form of urine. When it is too wet because of taking in too much damp-producing food, such as sweets, dairy products, and refined carbohydrates, it becomes sodden and swampy, like a saturated field. People with a strong spleen system have a lot of physical energy; those with a weak spleen feel tired and depleted.

Your center also governs which thoughts and memories you pay attention to and which you let go. Just as it separates what your body needs from what it doesn't in the digestive tract, your center takes in thoughts and experiences, digests and analyzes them, and then discards what is not necessary and nourishing.

A healthy center receives thoughts and then induces action on those thoughts or lets them go. But an unhealthy center may not process these thoughts properly, causing mental reflections to become stuck "overthinking." The Chinese believe that overthinking, which includes excessive thought, studying, concentrating, memorizing, pensiveness, worrying, and brooding, can, over time, weaken the spleen and inhibit the optimal functioning of its energy processes. This is why excessive worry causes digestive disturbances such as stomach ulcers and irritable bowel syndrome—too much information clogs up our mind and obstructs the earth energy flowing through our center, preventing us from making proper decisions, and causing disharmony. Always return to your center where pure awareness resides.

🌻 The Healing Power of Dance and Song

Exercise contributes to the proper functioning of the spleen energies. But I don't only mean the kind of exercise you do in a gym, like running on a treadmill or riding a stationary bike. The kind of exercise I'm referring to is expressive movement that comes from within—dancing to the song inside you.

Dancing is healing. At Fertile Soul retreats we practice free, vibrant, creative movement. I encourage you, too, to dance, drum, sing, and move to express your innermost self and become an instrument of a greater song. While you dance you will resonate with life and sing a song no one else can sing. As the Persian mystic poet Rumi said:

> *You are a song, a wished-for song.*
> *Move to the center,*
> *Towards the sky and wind,*
> *Towards silent knowing.*

Accept the wished-for song that you are. Then sing not only with your voice but with your heart and soul and spirit. Until you find the link and open the path between all the sacred parts of you, you will be singing a made-up song, someone else's song. But when you let life live through you, you will sing your own.

Voices express the words we think. Do you like your voice? If you don't, it may be telling you something important about yourself. For example, when I was a child I constantly felt lonely and in emotional pain. My voice had a quaver to it, which embarrassed me horribly. That quaver expressed my pain and unhappiness. At first I tried to cover it up by staying silent, but eventually I learned that alcohol and medication made it go away. Once the medication wore off, though, my sadness and hurt, my soul's song, were once again revealed in the quavering of my voice.

When I went deep within myself to my personal place of darkness, I heard what my voice had been telling me all along: that I was sensitive and compassionate and in unbearable emotional pain, which I was trying to hide. And when I accepted this aspect of my being, the pain started to fall away, all on its own. Acknowledging the makeup of my source allowed me to accept and let go of my pain. Though my voice still quavers from time to time, especially if I'm nervous or overstressed, now I have compassion for the little girl who developed that quaver as the result of a distressing childhood. By listening to the song of my voice and my soul I healed myself.

The Healing Power of Sound

Have you ever noticed your mind overthinking, producing chattering thoughts? Have you ever found yourself reflecting those thoughts by talking incessantly? Just as most people don't listen to people who talk constantly, most of us don't listen to our own chattering thoughts—sometimes we even try to drown them out. My husband, for example, after a trying day, used to try to drown out the thoughts spinning around in his head by listening to loud music and sitting in front of a blaring television. But inner chatter is telling us that something is wrong. It's important to accept and release the cause of the imbalance; the renewed energy dissolves the noise in our way. Excessive talk is usually good only for hurling out opinions, making judgments, and announcing how we want to be perceived by the world. It is better to save our voices for our inner song, the only thing that truly matters.

Sound, like song, can also heal imbalanced earth energies and allow life to live through you. In fact, I often use sound during healing, meditative sessions with clients. To use sound to increase your well-being, find a tone inside your mind that represents your idea of what the Divine sounds like. For example, the sound Om represents God in some traditions. Let this tone resonate within your very being; change it if you need to so that the tone represents the Divine within your heart. Then use the sound as your own special prayer to the Divine and to heal yourself.

A thirty-year-old retreat patient of mine, Belinda, had a tragic history of being sexually abused by her father. Despite this, when her father become terminally ill just as she was trying to have a first child, she cared for him lovingly until he passed away. After her father died, Belinda's blood work told her doctor that she was in absolute, irreversible menopause—her FSH level was 150 (a reading over 50 indicates menopause). Knowing how much pain this situation caused Belinda, her neighbor lent her a healing bowl, with which she meditated daily. Each time she meditated, she rubbed a stick around the outside of the bowl's lip, causing the bowl to make a sound in tune with the energies of the kidneys, which represent the sexual energies. The following month, Belinda's FSH level was 7, indicating she was not in menopause, only in protective mode. She had healed herself.

The Healing Power of Caring for Yourself

Earth energies are caring and nurturing. Like the earth itself, these energies are centered, stable, grounded, and abundant, and they enable us to be kind, helpful, sweet, generous, and supportive, both to ourselves and to others. They help to sustain the momentum of other moving energies and also to draw others to us.

When earth energies are out of balance, people forget to support and love themselves; they lose themselves trying to please others. They have difficulty saying no. They resist change and cling to what they know. They become overburdened, both physically and mentally. They lack energy, and worry to the point of obsession. Physically, digestion becomes sluggish. Allergies and fluid retention are common. People with earth energy imbalances may crave starches and sweets. When the imbalance is severe, they may develop diabetes.

Imbalanced spleen energies can result in a total loss of self. People with this imbalance live for their spouses, parents, children, or friends. They become so good at taking care of the outside world that they forget how to take care of their sacred selves. Eventually, their internal protective mechanism—their immune system—can turn against them, and they can develop autoimmune diseases. While they see others as friends, they become their own enemies, and their cells reflect the internal battle.

Lananda developed a condition in which her body initiated an assault on her entire endocrine system, a condition known as panendocrinopathy, which caused most of her hormonal system to shut down. At the Fertile Soul retreat she learned that her issues centered around taking care of others at her own expense. I put her on a program in which she defined her boundaries and fiercely honored them while she ate healthy, organic foods fresh from the ground. Within eight months, Lananda's endocrine system completely returned to normal.

Unsticking Earth Energies

To mobilize and resolve stuck earth energies, there are a number of things you can do. As I said earlier, singing, dancing, and making joyous sounds that connect you with the Divine are important. But you also need to care for yourself. That involves developing self-confidence, seeking inner guidance, and following a routine of healthful nourishment and activity.

Eating mindfully

Earth energy imbalance leads to sugar craving. If you indulge the craving, the rise and fall in your blood sugar levels will negatively affect your kidneys and spleen and cause the release of stress hormones to deal with the imbalance. To bring spleen energies back in balance and lower blood sugar levels and stress, avoid eating simple sugar in all of its forms, including cake, candy, and pastries. Also curtail:

- ❀ Heavy, greasy foods
- ❀ Starches
- ❀ Fats
- ❀ Dairy products
- ❀ Pasta
- ❀ Wheat
- ❀ Rich sauces

You should also avoid eating any food that is ice cold, since your body needs to heat it up before it can utilize it. If you are interested in trying herbal remedies, ginseng (any kind) and astragalus teas are excellent spleen tonics. Find a good natural food store or talk to a Chinese-medicine pharmacist to get some good personal recommendations.

In addition to being mindful of the food you eat, pay attention to the entire eating process, from preparing your food to the last swallow and dab with the napkin. Many people eat either to fill the emptiness inside or to make their taste buds happy. But eating is really about fulfilling ourselves and acknowledging that life is an exchange of energy in the form of breath, thoughts, emotions, actions, and food.

To eat mindfully, chew every piece of food thoroughly. Gather as much saliva as you can with each mouthful and swallow deeply; when maximized and properly utilized, saliva can raise the glutathione level in the intestine, which lubricates healthy joint function. After you swallow a bite, think about where the food is going and connect with it inside your body as well.

Not long ago I had a profound and rejuvenating experience eating an orange. I had taken a ten-minute break from a harried day and retreated to my kitchen for something to eat; my energies were all stuffed between my ears and I couldn't find peace or access the wisdom within me. As I sat at the table, I did nothing but eat my orange. I held it. I felt its firm roundness and looked at the dimples in its skin. I connected with the orange and then I began to peel it.

As I unwrapped the gift, I inhaled the sprays of aroma that ignited my sense of smell. I looked mindfully at the naked orange as it lay before me, urging me to help the segments nature had prepared blossom into my nourishment. As I picked up the first segment, I noticed how it had a unique identity. I looked, I connected, I bit. Sprays of flavor shot throughout my mouth as I paid attention to how my saliva mingled with the juice. I swallowed. I looked at the remainder of the segment into which I had bitten and noticed the tiny packages of bound orange nectar, waiting to be a part of my next experience of bliss. I bit again. I savored the next bite as well, and continued until I was in tears. That orange was the best meal of my life, and after eating it I went back to work as if it were a new day. All it took was eating mindfully—by savoring that orange I savored life.

When we connect with the food we put into our mouths, we connect with the food's source as well as with our digestive system. Native people long ago even connected with the spirit of the animal whose meat they ate so that the spirit that gave the animal life would give them life as well. When we eat foods that were connected with the earth over a period of time, we receive their qi, which enhances our earth energies. Foods such as eggs from caged chickens that never walked on the ground contain much less qi and provide us with less energy. To eat mindfully and healthfully, you need to eat from nature—whole grains, fresh fruits and vegetables, and organic, compassionately killed animals—and avoid eating food that comes in a box.

Creating a sacred space
Maria came to her first Fertile Soul retreat after years of being unhappy with her life. She was at the point of giving up and had let her house go, as well as her health, her appearance, and her passion. At the retreat, I encouraged her to shift from despair to focus on the wild excitement of the unknown. I also talked to her about creating a sacred space in her home, full of abundance, joy, and light, where she could sit peacefully and happily and find and strengthen her center. Maria didn't consider herself artful or creative, though, and felt intimidated by the process, so I recommended that she start out small by decorating a window or a corner of a room. She did just that, purchasing several candles and placing them on the ledge above her bathtub—she had often envisioned pretty women bathing in candlelight, but she had never allowed herself to bask in the glow herself. After she arranged the candles, she decided a hanging fern would feel right in her bathroom, too. And not long after, her creative flow extended into her bedroom, where she redecorated with new,

brighter draperies and a comforter to match. Then she enrolled in a home-decorating course at her local community college and, after enlivening the rest of her home, apprenticed with a local decorator. The last I heard, Maria had opened a design studio and was joyfully leading a new life.

Connecting with your true self

When you look in the mirror, who is looking back at you? Do you like whom you see? To unblock your earth energies, don't look at what you perceive as flaws. Instead, look deeply into your eyes and try to connect with a sense of compassion and love. Look at yourself and notice everything that you like. Look for the real you under your exterior and keep looking until you see yourself for who you truly are.

Doing things just for you

In addition to eating mindfully, creating a sacred space, and connecting with your true self, you can also rebalance your earth energies by caring for yourself in other ways:

- Exercise by doing something you enjoy that combines movement with muscular effort.
- Change your environment, for example, by rearranging your furniture in a more pleasing way.
- Take up a hobby or a creative project that provides pleasure for you (not with the goal of impressing anyone else).
- Learn to say no without giving a reason or making an excuse.
- Use self-affirmations when you speak and in your thoughts: "I feel ... ," "I feel like ... ," "I like my ..."; even if you don't mean what you say at first, you will eventually.
- If you are trying to build a family or having issues with your role as mother, step back and evaluate which roles that

have to do with parenting are most important to you (for example, being part of a larger family, giving a child opportunities you never had, assuring you will never be alone).

❀ Go for a hike in nature. Look at the flowers and trees and magnificent life in the soil. Gaze at the stars at night. Connect with how you feel during different phases of the moon. Smell the changes in the air when the weather shifts.

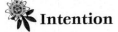 Intention

> *Accept the present and intend the future.*
>
> —DEEPAK CHOPRA

Worry, obsession, anxiety, and regret obstruct earth energy, squelching vitality. But when we are calm, aware, and open to all we can be, more energy flows through us.

The Chinese character for *yi*, 意, the soul of earth, or intention, represents the celestial vibration produced when the spirit is aligned with our actions. Having intention, or being directed and purposeful, brings us into alignment with our source and our spirit and lets our earth energies move freely. Having intention also allows thought to become belief, which can actually determine which of our inherited genes we activate and enables us to integrate past and future, hopes and dreams, and fears and passion within our center. Through you, the vessel, intention is made manifest, helping you to move forward with purpose, continue to transform yourself, and connect with your highest guidance to create the life you were meant to live.

As you learned earlier, though, it's important to first deal with the sludge within you in order to free up your internal space. Regret about the past and anxiety about the future disturb the spleen's function and prevent it from being balanced and stable, open to the present moment. So look without fear at those things in your life that are no longer working and use them to spur new growth and reach higher levels of being. Free yourself to let your earth energies release your full creative powers.

As the sprout is nourished by the earth, our wood's power to dream and create is acted upon through the spleen's energies of intention. Like our own Mother Earth, stable spleen energies enable us to harvest what we have planted. If you have planted negativity and fear, you will live in a fearful, negative world. If your beliefs reflect love and gratitude, you will live in a state of abundance.

The great half-woman, half-snake, Nu Wa,
created people from river mud.

She birthed and nursed our ancestors who
lived simply. When the Gods battled for land,
the world was nearing destruction. Nu Wa melted five
different colored jewels and
repaired all of heaven and earth.

—CHINESE LEGEND

Secret 5:
Let Go of Resistance

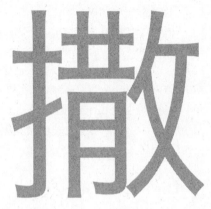

撒 *Release*

*There are two graces in breathing: drawing in air and
discharging it.*
*The former constrains, the latter refreshes: so mar-
velously is life mixed.*
*Thank God then when he presses you, and thank him
again when he lets you go.*

—JOHANN WOLFGANG VON GOETHE

One of the key principles of traditional Chinese medicine is to
not resist events, relationships, feelings—anything. That doesn't
mean that you should let yourself become a doormat, but rather
that you should be open and receptive to life in all its forms,
particularly to your own inner strength and wisdom. When you
no longer struggle to control the outcome of your life, you reduce

inner tension, express your true nature, and connect with the world around you.

When you receive and let go, you are following the motions of the universe and of nature—the tides, the birth and death of a star, the waxing and waning of the moon, the expanding and contracting of magma in the earth's center, the opening and closing of flower petals, the rise and fall of your chest as you breathe, the cycle of sleeping and waking up. All of life moves in and out, filling and emptying, naturally expanding to embrace the next level of existence.

The Metal Energies

The lung energies govern the lungs, skin, and the lungs' paired organ, the large intestine—the organs that enable us to breathe in and expel what we do not need. These energies, which are also called metal energies, magnetically attract atoms of chemical elements such as hydrogen and oxygen into the more complex molecular bonds that are necessary for organic life. The energies in the lower abdomen then magnetically pull these complex bonds into our core and allow the spirit to breathe.

The metal energies also connect with *po*, the corporeal soul that aligns with the ethereal soul to preside over physical being and regulate internal processes through the autonomic nervous system. As the chemical elements of air infuse us with the breath of life, po infuses us with our individual spirit, allowing us to see value in our emotions, feelings, outlook, and life. Po grasps life and represents our instinctual knowing, our sense of touch and being touched. Po is associated with beginnings and continuation and enables us to appreciate and revere each breath we take. It is also associated with the color white, the color of bones. Po represents the death of the dense self-centered ego, and the resurrection of the pure untainted self. Po allows us to say yes to life, and stays with us until it expires with our last breath.

Breathing, therefore, not only infuses our cells with life-giving oxygen, it connects us to all things and allows us to go to the depths of our feelings and our core. When we focus on breathing, we go to our foundation and connect with our spirit. In fact, in many ancient languages, breath and spirit are synonymous. I once read that indigenous Hawaiians described Europeans who reached their islands as "the men who pray without breathing" because it was unthinkable to them that people could connect with the Divine without employing their breath.

Taking in air, and with it po, our energies are enlivened by the sun and lifted high, just as the downward force of a bird's flapping wings allows it to rise into the sky. And when we exhale, we give back our breath to the universe to enable plants to survive. In between inhaling and exhaling lies the internal abyss, the source of contentment and connection to all of creation. As Rumi wrote in his poem "The Embryo":

> When the time comes for the embryo to receive the
>   spirit of life,
> At that time the sun begins to help.
> This embryo is brought into movement, for the sun
>   quickens it with spirit.
> From the other stars this embryo received only an
>   impression,
> until the sun shone upon it.
> How did it become connected with the shining sun in
>   the womb?
> By ways hidden from our senses:
> the way whereby gold is nourished,

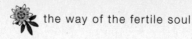

the way a common stone becomes a garnet and the
*   ruby red,*
the way fruit is ripened,
and the way courage comes to one distraught with fear.

We are born with a sense that we are the universe, that every-thing revolves around us. Then, as we grow, we realize we are individual entities and spend the rest of our lives developing our identities. We also form bonds—with our parents, siblings, part-ners, and friends—some of which we keep for life and some of which we let go. Like the coming and going of the air we breathe, we form and release friendships as we become different people ourselves. We learn about ourselves in relation to others when we take off our masks to reveal our soft inner selves.

This process of individuation, connection, and letting go, which is governed by the metal energies, involves risk. Forming bonds that may be relinquished exposes us to potential sadness and grief. But it also opens us up to new possibilities. As we do when we're dancing, we hold hands, let go, go back to the place from where we started, and clasp hands with another. When partners change, the dance becomes new again. And the dance enables us to find our true selves.

But the metal energies not only give us our sense of self; they eventually free us from the need to have others provide our sense of belonging. They help us to attach, separate, and gain an ever-widening relationship with the world—through friends, schools, church, career, and cultural organizations. As we become aligned higher and higher with the energy of the cosmos, our initial illusory separation from the Divine that began when we accepted our first breath comes full circle and we feel ourselves connected with every-thing and find the Divine everywhere, both within and without.

This return to the true self is associated with the energies of the fall: with the old giving way to await the emergence of the new. Though trees whose leaves lie on the ground appear dead, with patience, when warmth and light return, those trees will sprout again. Only death, whose contracting energies we so vehemently resist, allows new life to emerge. While it can be extremely painful to let part of your life fall away—some things that you simply don't want to let go—that release allows your powerful metal energies to raise you to new levels and bring new life and new possibilities.

Imbalanced Metal Energies

Metal energies protect us from the external environment. Deficient lung energies show up in the breath and skin. Allergies are a common finding in one whose lung energies are weak. So are respiratory ailments such as asthma, shortness of breath, chronic or recurring coughs, sinus infections, frequent colds, skin rashes, and hives. Since metal energies govern release, and thus the ability to defecate, imbalanced metal energies can also manifest in chronic constipation.

Metal energies that are not aligned and balanced can make you stiff and resistant, just like metal. The po grasps life itself, and when excessive metal energies are expressed, life can be grasped too tightly. People with imbalanced metal energies may spend undue effort trying hard to control themselves and everyone and everything in their lives. But, as many of us have learned, imposing control never works. Life is moving, not static, and although we can shape it, it cannot be controlled.

This goes against societal training, which, from the very first rules we are taught by our parents, teaches us to follow norms and laws determined by an external authority. So people come to believe that all things unwanted can be controlled. They try endlessly to control the conditions in their lives, and by doing so make things even worse than they are, because resistance causes contraction, not receptivity. For example, women who believe they are infertile contract themselves into a state of fear, sadness, and loss, making themselves less and less open to new life. At my Fertile Soul retreats, I continually see women who have tried everything to conceive a child. But the more they fight, the less receptive to life they become.

This resistance, this fierce struggle to command the coming of a child, is the first aspect I deal with at my fertility retreats. I work to help my patients let go and stop fighting, and open themselves to a receptive, expansive state. So many women who haven't been able to become pregnant finally do when they come to a state of acceptance and stop trying. That's why it's common for women to conceive after they've adopted a child. Letting go of the fight for a child lets them shift into a state of being that offers possibility and hope. Opening up inside and allowing life to breathe through you puts you in a place of balance and lets in creation, be it a child, a new way of living, a new dream, or a new project or career.

A fussy woman named Wanda once came to a retreat consumed with every little detail of every aspect of her life. She was a financial analyst and her inquiring, penetrating mind served her well in business but made her extremely intense and anxious. She was a self-described hypochondriac and wanted to know every detail about her body's symptoms, and thought her health care providers should give them to her. She was completely detached from her body and continually asking other people to provide answers for her: "Why does my cycle do this? Why is my blood this color? Why do I wake up at night to urinate?" She also had difficulty with the movement exercises I prescribe to help retreat-goers loosen up and release. Wanda had a rigid build, could make no sense of her body, and literally couldn't let go. She proclaimed, "I didn't come here to let go; I came here to get pregnant."

Wanda was slow to make progress, but eventually was able to let go a bit. During her time at the retreat she lightened up, was fun to be around, and became more open and receptive. But once she returned home, her anxiety seeped back in. She e-mailed me with new concerns: "I don't know when I ovulated. My period never came. My temperature never went down. Something is wrong!" When she took her worries to her local doctor, he confirmed that she was pregnant.

Physically Rebalancing Your Metal Energies

Taoists believe that during the process of receiving and letting go, the metal energies can fall out of balance, causing your spirit or soul to say no to life. Fortunately, there are several ways to realign your metal energies and restore balance to aid you in connecting to your highest level.

Detoxification

Keeping your metal energies pure and healthy requires taking in every breath deeply. It also requires eliminating the old in order to let new vital energy in. We release the old through exhalations, skin cells, sweat, tears, and feces. The intestines, skin, and lungs eliminate what no longer serves us, detoxifying the body's energies.

To help your skin eliminate the old, exfoliate your body daily with a skin brush or a dry washcloth. This process will, both literally and figuratively, shed your old skin so that promising new skin can appear. As you exfoliate, bring intention to the process. Being mindful to treat yourself gently, consider what you need to eliminate and brush it all away. Taking a sauna will also cleanse and detoxify your pores.

Having a healthy bowel movement each day is another important way your body eliminates toxins. Drinking plenty of water and eating plenty of roughage in fiber-rich fruits, vegetables, and grains will help to cleanse yourself of what you don't need and prevent toxins from being absorbed into your system. If you have trouble eliminating—many of the women I treat suffer from constipation—reduce the heat in your system, which can be the result of spicy foods and too much internal stress and tension. In addition to balancing the heat, try boiling rhubarb and prunes and drink their juice.

Also limit the food you eat in the evening. If you pack your gut right before bed, it will become overwhelmed with messages: to fill, extract water, and consolidate the residue; and to release the previous day's contents. Because the intestines rest at night, undigested food can rot in your gut and the toxic contents are sent into your bloodstream, making elimination much less efficient the next day.

Self-massage

Skin sweats in order to lower body temperature. It also senses pain to keep us away from danger. These automatic responses do a great deal to prevent harmful substances from entering our bodies.

To be mindful of the importance of your skin, massage yourself as part of your daily or nightly self-care routine. Traditional Chinese medicine believes massage is a beautiful way to thank your body. Take baths and follow them by massaging yourself with natural lotions scented with soothing essential oils, such as lavender. Let your skin know that you are aware of and appreciate what it does for you by massaging your face, scalp, hands, and feet. Be aware of how your touch feels and indulge in its comfort.

Mentally and Emotionally Rebalancing Your Metal Energies

Detoxifying your body will do much to enable you to take in life-giving energy and release substances that are not good for you. But you also need to enable your mind and spirit to release attachments that are toxic to you. Ask yourself each day, What am I willing to let go of? Identifying unhealthy attachments to things, people, work, or life situations will allow you to evaluate whether you need to enforce boundaries, adjust the situation, or leave it altogether.

Crying is one way we release attachments. When we are sad or grieving, our bodies contract, the lungs and chest tighten, and this pressure is released in a cry or moan. Failing to surrender to the need to cry and let go results in a lower state of energy in which we haven't the strength to power ourselves upward.

Denial and resistance inhibit the proper expansion of lung energies and are counter to the spirit's upward and outward direction. While it is natural and necessary to mourn significant losses, mourning that continues too long puts you at odds with yourself, preventing you from establishing a higher order, which can be achieved only through surrender. If you cannot accept external reality, then your internal wisdom begins to unravel. A split develops between perception and reality, which exhausts vitality and creates havoc.

To prevent this from happening, ancient Chinese societies decreed that when a father died, his son was allowed three days of total immersion in grief, during which time he wept uninterrupted as he cared for his father's body. After the three days had passed, the intense grieving period ended and life went on (although the mourning period could last one year). The lesson of this is that after immersing ourselves in our grief it is essential to then let it go.

One of the most potent ways to heal grief is soul-to-soul communication in which we connect with another person's release through tears. As rivers flow into the ocean, our own affliction can be relieved by aligning ourselves with the waterways of another. Have you ever felt like crying when you truly felt someone else's grief? When we join our tributary of tears to another, the soul is touched and healed.

I witness this incredible form of healing at every Fertile Soul retreat. As women who are going through similar heartaches share their stories, dramatic healing takes place. As they see each other, care about each other, and share their pain, their own pain lessens a bit. Though each of them may feel broken, when they connect with another person going through similar pain, they still see the other person as whole—and then can't help seeing themselves that way, too.

Emotional healing comes through surrender, when you allow yourself to be taken to that unknown place where you have no control. There you let the pressure within your depths work on you, transforming your rough edges and transforming your carbon potential into a diamond. Complete abandonment provides utter release and freedom, actually restructuring you and enabling you to live according to a pure state where your energies actually vibrate at a higher level.

Sophia, an Eastern European immigrant and only child, saw her grandfather die when she was six and lost her father when she was ten. At a retreat she revealed how her mother, who barely survived World War II, clutched Sophia to her tightly, hardly letting her breathe. Sophia felt joined to those who had died, and lived her own life unhappily, feeling dead inside. At the retreat, we worked on restoring her po using her acceptance and release of death with acupuncture, intention, and journaling. After she surrendered to the deepest grief she had ever felt, she became able to embrace life at last.

The Metal Energies' Transforming Power

Just as metal can be reshaped by intense heat, the metal energies can combine with other energies to enable transformation. When metal, water, wood, and earth combine and are allowed to gestate deep within you, they enable you to reach your highest self. Through the process of alchemy these energies mold you into a new state of being.

But you can't force or control this interaction—it comes through release. And its power doesn't manifest on the surface. Just as metals form deep within the earth, transformation takes place deep within. There, the intense pressures of life do their work—suffering and pain are turned to awareness and enlightenment. The highest, purest creations come from the strongest pressures of life. In my own case, learning to let go of the immense suffering I went through is what enabled me to reach the ecstatic heights I later experienced. It was the fuel for my transformation.

The transformative process begins by knowing yourself and loving your source—deeply.

❀ **Water**—You must accept yourself, wrinkles, warts, shadow aspect, and all. From this state of being, the desire to create, to become, grows.

❀ **Wood**—You hold the vision of what you desire to create. Then, to enable creativity, you align your love of self with thoughtful intention and action.

❀ **Earth**—What actions do you need to take to align yourself with this focused intent? And then, by letting go and not resisting, you let life mold you into a new and abundant state of being.

❀ **Metal**—Surrender to what is. You don't run or hide. You release the old so a new order can be established.

❀ **Fire**—Open up to your highest aspect of being, your spirit.

The downward energy of metal is what propels us upward.

In this way, you follow in the footsteps of one of the highest mythical representations in Chinese mythology, the Queen Mother of the West, Xi Wang Mu, goddess of the ultimate yin. The Queen Mother resides where the earth turns away from the sun, representing the death of all things that no longer serve. She symbolizes the aspect of the Divine feminine that lets old habits die, releases inappropriate partners, and stops harmful life interactions. She also represents the death of the physical form when we are finished with this earthly vehicle.

Phoebe was a model whose greatest fear was losing her youth and beauty. Whenever she saw a wrinkle, she saw death sneaking up on her. The spiritual teacher Bhagavan Das says, "When you can't remember God, remember death. It will bring you there." After I talked with Phoebe, she decided to face her fear of death directly and began to visit a nursing home, spending time every week with those who had no family. After doing this for some time, Phoebe realized it wasn't death she feared; it was a new phase in her life that she was afraid of. Who would she be without her looks? Realizing this made her feel shallow, which

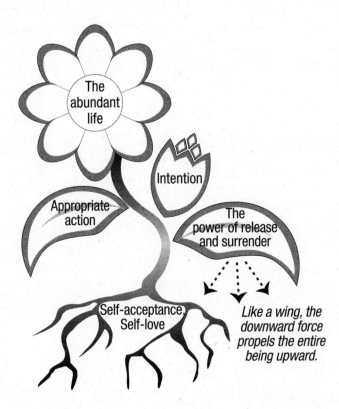

The abundant life

Intention

Appropriate action

The power of release and surrender

Self-acceptance, Self-love

Like a wing, the downward force propels the entire being upward.

she didn't like. She worked on creating a newer, better self by visiting the home almost every night, reading to the elders, combing their hair, and making them feel loved and cared for. In that way, she also loved and cared for herself.

Finding Your Own Way

Until you become aware of and connected to your source, soul, and spirit, you may rely on your connections with others to feel secure and stable. But when you understand from where you came and who you are, you can walk the path you were meant to walk, majestic in your solitude. As Albert Einstein said:

I am truly a lone traveler and have never belonged to my country, my friends, or even my immediate family with my whole heart; in the face of all these ties, I have never lost a sense of distance and a need for solitude, feelings which increase through the years.

Eventually, our spiritual path narrows to where two cannot walk abreast. We walk alone, yet through our breath we are connected to our inner stillness and aware of our connection to everything around us. The electromagnetic force created by lung energies interacting with source energies allows us to walk upright, aware, stable, and strong. Through surrender and acceptance, though it seems our very foundation is being shaken, we allow our essence below the surface to break through and become a fountain of support, love, and purpose in the world.

I accept the universe.

—Margaret Fuller

Secret 6:
Live from Your Joy Rather Than Your Fear

生 *Emergence*

And the day came when the risk to remain tight in
 a bud
Was more painful than the risk it took to blossom.

— ANAÏS NIN

You've learned in the previous chapters that the water energies represent the full expression of self. You've also seen that wood energies stand for the energies associated with change and opportunity. The earth energies bring it all together in your core. And the metal energies signify releasing all that is inappropriate or damaging so that you can live as your true self. The fire, or heart, energies are the energies of emergence, which allow you to blossom from a tightly bound bud to a full, unrestricted, radiant flower.

When, as so many of us have been trained, fear is used as a guiding emotion, it blocks access to this full expression of joy. With the many advantages of a fruitful society also comes a tendency for us to sign over our personal power and be guided by external authority. This leads to many common, paralyzing fears: fear of not being good enough, fear of what people think, doubts about your own inner knowing, and so forth. Through practice, even deeply ingrained negative thought habits can be replaced with the infinitely more powerful thoughts founded in love, allowing for your natural expansion and creativity.

Fire Energies

The heart energies arise from the center of your chest and power you to immense vitality and infinite potential. Traditional Chinese medicine views the heart as the home of the spirit. As it pumps blood, it circulates the spirit throughout the physical being. When fear, anger, and grief are transformed through intention, spirit moves unobstructed through the body, allowing us pure connection with all things. When our heart energies are balanced and aligned, we connect with the world through love.

As you can see in the following horizontal-vertical grid, the heart energies take you to the zenith of your existence, crowning the acceptance at the base of the grid and the horizontal "doing" energies of wood and metal around the central pivot of earth's knowing. At this apex you live as pure spirit and in peace.

Signs of Imbalanced Heart Energies

The heart governs the spirit, so its manifestations show up in the psyche. If you are prone to heart palpitations, anxiety, agita-

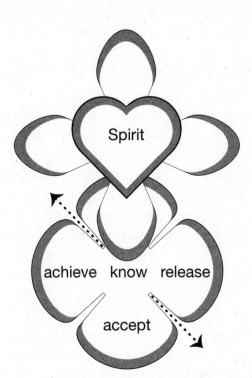

tion, or restlessness, or if you fidget, flush easily, are frequently impatient, lack vitality, have nightmares, or can't sleep deeply throughout the night, you likely have deficient heart energies. Because the spirit is contained in blood, deficient heart energies are also evidenced in conditions in which blood moves less freely through the vessels, such as blood stasis, a condition that develops as we age. They can also be seen in diseases that make you prone to blood clots, heart attacks, embolisms, and strokes.

In the system of traditional Chinese medicine, the heart encompasses consciousness, the highest aspect of the mind that contains the insight by which the will of heaven is known. Therefore, if your heart energies are blocked or imbalanced, your emotions may become unstable or shattered, causing you to lose your barometer for reality. For example, you can become convinced that you have nothing to contribute to life and be unable to live vivaciously.

Imbalanced heart energies manifest either as excessive or insufficient energy. For example, when someone burns the candle at both ends, becoming hyperactive, grandiose, or wild, the fire energies are too hot and cause them to burn out of control. Excessive fire energies can also affect the psyche, causing disturbed, manic, or even psychotic behavior—a state Chinese medicine paradoxically refers to as too much joy. This doesn't mean too much happiness; it means overindulgence of excitement, entertainment, ego gratification, constantly doing too much, socializing too much, spending too much time talking on the phone, watching television, or listening for too many hours to loud music. All this doing doesn't allow room for other energies that are needed for balance. The result is an internal void that is never filled, but which can sometimes be temporarily masked by excessive activity.

Insufficient fire energies, on the other hand, can result in depression, a lack of joy or passion, agitation, restlessness, and a search for worldly, rather than internal, fulfillment. Insufficient fire energies can also result in restless, interrupted sleep. The traditional Chinese medicine system explains that when the heart finds no inner anchor, the spirit can find no rest and wanders aimlessly throughout the night.

Activating the Divine Spark

When source energy becomes the basis of our actions, we activate our own Divine spark and live authentically. When source, soul, intention, and spirit are aligned, we spiral upward to reside in the highest plane of existence, that of unconditional love. In this state we don't choose what or who is worthy of our love, we simply love because it is our very nature—we *are* love. We live in abundance and joy, and extend the inherent ecstasy and bliss of life.

The energies of the heart are the most potent of all the life energies. The electromagnetic charge of the brain can be detected about twelve inches outside the perimeter of the skull but the energies of the heart can be picked up about twelve feet away from the person emitting them. When we are unhindered by the restrictions of fear, anger, worry, and grief, there is no limit to how far the heart energies can reach. Because the heart is such a powerful organ, the Chinese see it as the empress of the entire being, served by all the other energies. It rules from its throne deep within our chest, connecting us to every other spiritual current and supporting our

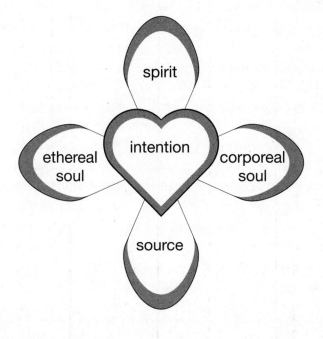

spirit's highest work—to give unconditional love to ourselves, everyone, and everything.

Rebalancing the Heart Energies

So how do we keep the heart energies open, balanced, and moving? By taking care of the other four energies—those of the kidneys, liver, spleen, and lungs. Those organs receive and interact, enabling the heart energies to give. That means that if your inner needs aren't met through the other four energy systems, your heart won't be able to pour out love.

Feeling gratitude and reverence is another way to keep the heart energies flowing. Yet, because we work hard for what we achieve, have, and eat, we tend to feel entitled, rather than grateful, for all the things in our lives. When we are able to feel and express gratitude for what we have, things get even better and creativity in all forms abounds. Being grateful keeps us open, receptive, and full of joy, and lets us give ourselves completely to life.

Each day, first thing in the morning, I take a few minutes to connect with life and express the energies of my heart. Just before I get out of bed, when my awareness starts coming into focus, my natural tendency is to rush into the concerns of the day and forget the real reason for living. So, before I allow myself to get out of bed, I connect with the inherent joy of life. Keeping my eyes closed, I quiet my mind and bring my awareness deep inside my chest and my heart. Doing this for just a few moments puts the rest of the day into proper perspective and, no matter what deadlines I have or what dramas arise, I continue to experience the joy of being alive.

Many women find keeping a gratitude journal to be another way to tap into feelings of love and appreciation. It's as simple as writing lists of things that you're grateful for: a person, a day, your work or family, or even your current surroundings. Start with easy topics and then see if you can find things that you're grateful for in more challenging relationships. Remember to consider the basic things that are so easy to take for granted. For example, where would we be without running water and electricity? On days when you feel less connected to your heart energies, looking through your journal will remind you of the many things that you are grateful for, enabling you to easily reconnect.

Body movement is another way to align energy. As discussed earlier, dancing lets you move to your own song and know your true inner nature. Dancing also balances the heart energies and helps you to live with excitement, passion, affection, and enthusiasm. When I conducted a retreat in India a couple of years ago, in fact, a yogi told us, "Women open up through dance." So move to your own beat. Dance into your temple.

In addition to dancing, try to be mindful about the many types of other movements you make throughout the day, and express and take pleasure from them whether it's painting, playing a guitar, walking, working out, biking, dancing, planting a flower garden, or making dinner. Our bodies were meant to move and every movement is an opportunity for pleasure.

To balance your fire energies and find stability and calm, it is also important to stay nourished and eat healthfully. Drink plenty of liquids and avoid overindulging in hot, spicy, or drying foods such as fiery Mexican, Indian, or Thai foods. Avoid coffee, caffeine, natural or artificial stimulants, and, of course, tobacco. Eat foods that nourish the blood and the yin, such as mung beans and beets. Several supplements, such as omega-3 fatty acids, pycnogenol, grape seed, pine bark, and bilberry extracts, can support smooth blood flow. Talk to a naturopath or other person knowledgeable in herbs and supplements to explore what might help you.

It is also important to take time for yourself, to go within for solitude and restitution, and to preserve your boundaries. This includes not feeling obligated to take on other people's burdens and refusing to let anyone else tell you how to live your life. Every day, make time for rest and deep relaxation. Practice the meditative breathing exercises taught throughout this book, especially before going to bed. During the day, practice expressing yourself and speaking your truth.

From your sense of the Divine, practice loving unconditionally. Ordinary love is rooted in desire and satisfaction, but Divine love has no boundaries and no conditions—nothing stands in its way. There is a difference between unconditional love and need. For example, if you can't love your husband or partner when he betrays you, that isn't love; it's need, need for another person's love in order to feel whole. Need is based in the other organs, not the heart. Need is an inward movement; love is an outward expression, like forgiveness. Yet, love isn't only something we exchange, it is what we are; and when we know this, we radiate it in all our encounters, even to those we don't particularly like.

Most love in this world is conditional and requires love in return. One of the most conditional relationships is that of the traditional husband-and-wife arrangement: I will love you and spend my life with you, but you in return must love me and be devoted to me and agree with me and support my desires and wishes. Love between a parent and child is the next most conditional relationship: I will love you and take care of you, but you in turn must love me and respect me and do what I tell you to do; you must receive gratefully all the love I give you, all the education and opportunities I bestow upon you, and you must perform and become a respectable young lady or gentleman in return.

But true unconditional love requires nothing in return, not even consideration. The trick to this: you have to love yourself unconditionally as well. When you realize that your longing for love can always be satisfied by the devine you, it releases your dependence on others and your need to control them in order to feel good. You may still need to express emotions about the behavior of those close to you, and adjust your own, but these actions do not alter the state of love. If you'd like to love purely, ask yourself if there is anyone for whom you can't feel love. Write down his or her name and journal about the feelings you have surrounding him or her. There is usually another emotion like fear, anger, worry, jealousy, or grief that inhibits the ability to love. Pray for or meditate on this person once per day for two weeks, asking that he or she be forgiven, and that all good things come their way. And then, see if you can send them love.

I try to parent my children by example, not through instruction. My children see me living my own passion—I have released them of the burden of having me live through them. I give them limits and try to guide them and be there for them, but I don't feel I own them and I do not need them to perform for me. What they accomplish will be their own and whatever it is, I will be proud of them. When I am anchored and healthy I am able to extend my love and goodwill without expecting return. And they can live freely. Children naturally want to do well for themselves, their friends, parents, and teachers. They learn a deep sense of independence when they follow role models rather than act out of fear of not meeting someone else's expectations. And they approach life with an inner directive, an inherent sense of responsibility for their own actions and consequences.

Relationships with animals are a wonderful way to stimulate feelings of unconditional love. Petting a cat or dog can immediately flood you with love. Nature can also do this: take time to appreciate how the wind blows through the trees, the way the air smells after a rain shower. Appreciating fully and purely is the same as unconditional love, allowing you to connect with life and joy.

Susan was a sweet, authentic woman who enjoyed the life she was leading, sharing it with two cats and a dog. Then she fell in love and married a man who was the only son of Greek immigrants, who felt it was his duty to produce a child to carry on the family name. But this wasn't Susan's path—her body, mind, and soul rejected participating in the process. When she came to a retreat, Susan had suffered through many in vitro procedures and had not become pregnant. She had, however, developed a life-threatening autoimmune disease.

As I worked with Susan, she discovered she had adopted a false identity for her husband and that she was not living her own truth. Her real passion was not to mother a child but to care for animal habitats in the wild. As she came into the strength of her own intention, Susan separated from her husband and found great joy on her new path. She also rekindled her relationship with her sister, who shared Susan's interest in working with animals. Susan also eventually rekindled her relationship with her husband, who found during the separation that Susan was his true love and that he belonged at her side, rather than meeting the obligations that his parents had laid on him. As she healed her life issues, she was able to wean herself off steroids as her autoimmunity went into remission.

Breaking Open, Not Breaking into Pieces

The heart has an amazing capacity to heal. After experiencing a heart attack the heart can recover and the person can go back to living an active life. When the heart is damaged in spiritual terms, from being jilted or losing a loved one or a dream, it can also recover—by being broken open rather than being broken into pieces.

Tragic situations can wound a heart and break it into pieces, which a person then spends the rest of her life trying to put back together, a goal hampered by an attitude of victimization and identity with a negative self-definition: I am an abuse victim, a child of an alcoholic, a mother against drunk drivers, an infertile woman. But trying to patch heart fragments back together requires a person to constantly relive the terrible story over and over, prolonging the pain of past suffering.

The alternative to this devastation is to let your heart be broken open, allowing true healing to take place. It is human nature to distract ourselves. Within the heart is the place the Buddhists call "the place of no hope," which may also be described as a place of no expectation that things will be different. While you may think that healing can't occur without the possibility of hope for something else, that is precisely when healing occurs—when there is no outside story to take you away from the present reality. Just as pure love is unconditional, pure hope is unconditional. The highest place of hope is not hoping for anything in particular, but to simply be present and to feel life in its completeness, no matter the circumstances. It is deep acceptance; it is trust and surrender at the same time.

To prepare for your heart to be opened, let what happens happen. Don't fight what is. Don't become the story, the drama, or the crisis. Allow. Stay fully and attentively present in the moment. You may still have fear, anxiety, anger, and hurt feelings, but your heart is open, able to heal and help others receive love as well.

Monique was an only child and knew she could have anything she wanted. When she grew up she became a legal aid lawyer and married a handsome man. After both her parents died, Monique rooted herself in her husband, but he was unfaithful to her. When she came, devastated, to a retreat, she was looking for a way to find a safe place for her roots to settle and for her to heal.

At all the Fertile Soul retreats, I use a therapeutic poetry exercise in which the women meditate and draw forth intention, then draw cards from a bowl. On each card is a single word, which the women string together to create their own poetry. Monique drew the words "roots," "fertile," and "sister." With those words, her healing began. She wrote, "I have found my fertile soul, I have found my true roots, and I have placed them within the nourishing love of my new fertile soul sisters." Monique continued to write healing poetry to help others heal, too. She had found a safe place to take root and a way to express and receive love.

Healing Yourself

Any man or woman who has the courage to overcome the limits of the mind can attain the state of universal motherhood. The love of awakened motherhood is a loving compassion not only for one's own children but for all people, animals, plants, rocks, and rivers. It is a love extended to all nature's beings. For one who has awakened to true motherhood, every creature is his or her child. Such love, such motherhood is divine Love, which is God.

—Amma Chi

One part of the work I do focuses on helping women discover their creative, fertile power before their children come to them. If women heal themselves before they become mothers, they live happier lives themselves and are able to create a better world for their children.

I began to learn this myself when one of my own babies was just a few weeks old. A visiting friend and I were having a deep talk about being daughters and mothers. As I held my daughter and looked at her absolute perfection, I got so choked up over the love I felt for my baby girl that I started to cry. I connected with my sorrow in not feeling loved in the same way I loved her. As I wept, I realized that this was connected to my intense need to have a child of my own. I was parenting the hurt and broken parts of myself through my child and the intense love I felt for my daughter was the very same love I had always been missing. Breaking open in this way and becoming aware of this fact created a conduit through which I was able to heal. The experience also made me realize the burden I might have placed on my daughter if I required her to fill my need for love, and hadn't healed my pain myself.

Do you know the old adage that we can't love others fully until we love ourselves? I think this is especially true when we're trying to become parents. I know that I couldn't fully parent my children until I was emotionally whole and loved myself. When I was trying to become pregnant, I took care of myself like never before. But once I had given birth, my sound wellness practices went out the window. I had gotten healthy in order to have a child, but I hadn't been motivated to have a healthy me.

The ingrained urge to care for myself through others still comes out in my interactions with my children. When Kyra decided not to go to a school dance, I panicked because I saw myself at her age, feeling lonely and rejected. But before I imposed my vicarious needs on her I was able to remember that she was Kyra, not me, and she was OK—she just didn't want to dance this particular dance. Whenever I approach her through the eyes of my own fear she gets annoyed with me and I have to come back to reality and realize that I still have some inner work to do. I choose not to mother from a stance of weakness, from what I didn't get as a child.

A mother who approaches her children from a place of wisdom rather than a conditional place of need, fear, or control, will foster a healthy independence in them. From the state of "universal motherhood," the difference between parenting and living someone else's life becomes clear. Just as I never belonged to my mother, my children don't belong to me. They were given life by their source, not by my desire. And I am no more whole because of my children than I was when I imagined that their absence was the source of my emptiness. As the great philosopher-poet Kahlil Gibran said in his seminal work, *The Prophet*:

> *Your children are not your children.*
> *They are the sons and daughters of Life's longing for*
>   *itself.*
> *They come through you but not from you,*
> *And though they are with you, yet they belong not to*
>   *you.*
> *You may give them your love but not your thoughts,*
> *For they have their own thoughts.*
> *You may house their bodies but not their souls,*
> *For their souls dwell in the house of tomorrow,*

Which you cannot visit, not even in your dreams.
You may strive to be like them, but seek not to make
  them like you.
For life goes not backward nor tarries with yesterday.
You are the bows from which your children as living
  arrows are sent forth.
The archer sees the mark upon the path of the
  infinite,
And He bends you with His might that His arrows
  may go swift and far.
Let your bending in the Archer's hand be for
  gladness;
For even as He loves the arrow that flies, so
He loves also the bow that is stable.

You are the bow. The Divine is the archer. And you are being bent with might. Don't resist the tension—allow life to mold you. Though it may seem at times that you don't have the capacity to bear the challenge, you can and you will. You'll do it by forgiving, by letting go, by finding the invincible strength within your own heart. You'll do it by taking care of every aspect of yourself that feels empty or neglected. Acknowledge any inner emptiness, feel the feelings, breathe into the peace of your inner void, and surrender to it. Your inner stillness will become your greatest source of power when you detach yourself from hitting the mark and pay attention only to what you can control: the pull of the arrow, the direction, and the release.

What are the arrows you wish to let fly? A song? A way to help others? A new career? Higher education? How far are you willing to bend to the Divine archer? Your kidney energies govern the tension behind the bow and how far the arrow can fly. How deeply are you willing to look inside yourself?

What is on hold and needs to be unleashed—an unfinished project? A dormant profession? The liver energies allow the string to be released so the arrow can soar. What awakens the creative urge inside you and how will you encourage that urge so that it may be released? The spleen energies govern your intention or your aim in life. Where are your aspirations directed, and where are your sights set? The lung energies represent the target itself. Can you pay attention to the arrow rather than the target? Can you release the object of your desire so you aren't overly attached to the mark? And once you release the arrow, can you surrender to the process of the heart itself and enjoy the spiritual journey, soaring along the path of the infinite?

Denai never wanted children. She was a free spirit who lived life fully. When she was about forty, she became pregnant, an unplanned event that resulted in an early miscarriage. To her surprise, the miscarriage devastated her. She came to the Fertile Soul retreat to achieve another pregnancy, but soon recognized that it wasn't a baby that she desired. We checked what the pull of Denai's bow really represented, and redirected her aim. She described this as an awakening: "Something deep inside of me shifted. But the need wasn't for a child. The process in my uterus caused the emergence of a need to express myself from within my very bones." When Denai let go, she felt like the pregnancy made her aware of a great creative power within her. She tried her hand at an old love, writing, and wrote a workbook for women on how to express the joy of life. She allowed herself to be bent with gladness, and by trusting the divine archer she learned to live and love from the deep authentic place in her soul.

✳ Meditation to Open the Heart and Bring the Spirit Home

To tap into your own well of boundless opportunity, practice this meditation to open your heart and release your fear.

Begin by breathing into your chest, expanding and contracting your ribs and diaphragm so your lungs can fill and empty. Follow this movement; become mesmerized by this movement. Then turn your awareness deep into your heart. Feel the place where your breath meets the pulsing of your heart. Still yourself until you can connect with the breath above and the heartbeat below. Keep going deeper into the void within the center of your heart. Go as deep as you can and feel the stillness that connects you to the entire universe.

In the depths of the emptiness, bring your awareness again to your beating heart, which is constant and steadfast, always there for you and waiting to express its abundance. Envision your heart as the empress on her throne, with all the other organ systems supporting her. Listen calmly and quietly to what she needs from you. Be patient and give it time. It takes time and practice to establish rapport so the empress trusts you. She will tell you what she understands you are ready to hear. She knows what's best. Trust her rule.

As you practice this meditation, continue to connect with your heart as you go through your day. When you see an opportunity, quiet your mind, bring your awareness deep within your chest, and listen to and appreciate your heartbeat. Feel its constant, reverberating beat and the love it is sending.

Love is the Water of Life.
Drink it down with heart and soul.

—RUMI

Secret 7:
Use Your Emotions to Revitalize Your Life

信 *Trust Your Emotions*

*Praise and blame, gain and loss, pleasure and sorrow
come and go like the wind.*
*To be happy, rest like a great tree in the midst of
them all.*

— ACHAAN CHAA

According to traditional Chinese medicine, emotions are simply reactions to the environment and, no matter what they are, they're good and natural and serve us best when they are experienced, expressed, and let go. A complete range of emotions is necessary for responding to the world and for connecting with ourselves as well as with others, but, like blocked qi, unexpressed or squelched emotions cause obstructions in the body and create resistance that wreaks havoc on perspective, relationships, and health.

When you have a thought, it is usually accompanied by an emotion, which is a response to an event or your interpretation of an event. Emotions are literally energy in motion. They carry charges that affect the body: joy and elation are felt as high, positive charges and anger and fear are felt as low, negative charges.

When these charges aren't able to move—say, for example, when something isn't working out the way you want it to—they can become stuck in the body, a tight knot of bound energy. This tightness becomes a source of stress and drains away energy. To release bound-up emotions, you need to open up the fist that is holding them tight, releasing the emotion's grip physically, mentally, and emotionally. The hypothalamus, our main endocrine control center in the brain, is an extremely sensitive relay station for transmitting emotionally charged messages from the brain to the pituitary gland and on to the body's endocrine glands, impacting almost all of our hormonal and physical responses.

The more bound up in layers of thought emotions become, the more deeply they are stuck inside. Emotions such as guilt, shame, jealousy, and regret may become wrapped in a knot of negativity that has to be untied layer by layer with consistent work and plenty of patience. Fortunately, no matter how strong these emotions are, they can be released and gently let go, restoring health and harmony.

How Emotions Affect Our Organs

Health comes from returning to stillness. When our emotions are triggered, they are like trees moving in the wind. If the trees resist the wind's force, they can break and fall. But if they move with the wind, they become part of the music of the universe, eventually returning to their original, still position, healthy and alive. Like trees, we must experience the force of our emotions and move with them. Not resist, but yield. Then we must express the emotions, let them go, and return to a state of balance.

This is the natural way. A tree does not say, "I don't want this wind today; perhaps if I stand still enough, it won't move me." But most of us would like to deny the wind. We don't want to experience changes that evoke powerful emotions such as sadness and anger; we want to control our surroundings in an effort to experience only pleasant emotions and make our own happy music.

All of us need emotions, *all* of our emotions, to respond appropriately to our world and to relate to ourselves and others. To prevent suffering caused by squelching or harboring excess emotion, we need to flow with the natural way and always return to a state of balance and calm.

When our environment calls for a response, it produces tension that evokes an emotion, each of which is governed by one of the elements. When a response is called for, the qi of the particular organ system reacts to the situation. In the Chinese medical text the *Neijing*, the Yellow Emperor asks his physician, Qi Bo, to explain which emotions are governed by which organs and what happens as a result of resisting the emotions or hanging onto them for too long. Qi Bo's answers, which I enlarge on here, will help you understand the link between emotions and well-being.

When there is fear, qi descends

The kidneys, through the adrenal glands, govern the instinct for self-preservation, the most basic energy for staying alive. Their job is to stand guard, pay attention, and look out for danger. Normally their energies promote caution, self-restraint, prudence, and withdrawal, but when fear dominates someone's life, their qi plummets to near collapse. This happens because the kidneys' water energies, which draw down and condense under proper, free-flowing circumstances, are shocked by fear into sudden contraction, preventing energies from moving upward at all. An acute example of this process is someone experiencing a severe fright and wetting themselves. If fear continues to rule and caution and restraint become a way of life, these energies become pathologic and retreat too far in and down, eventually severing the axis between the heart and the kidneys. The festering energies then create a void in the heart and spirit, which fills with timidity, uncertainty, agitation, and a lack of vitality. Physically, this void can lead to symptoms like anxiety or heart palpitations.

A criminal lives this way, in a constant state of panic, afraid of being caught. You may sometimes live this way, too, and feel the damaging results. To overcome such harmful emotions, it's important to distance yourself from them. Reflective thought, like a mirror that reveals what's around the corner, lets you see more clearly and objectively, making the space in which you can develop the courage to face your fears.

When there is anger, the qi rises up

Healthy wood, or liver, energies are fresh and alive and necessary to overcome resistance. But when these energies are blocked or imbalanced, resistance—to what is or is supposed to be—is fueled, causing frustration and stress, because we rarely can change the way things are. Frustration produces aggravation, resentment, and anger. Anger thrusts up and out—this is why you can feel people's anger even if they don't express it.

When anger, either excessive or suppressed, obstructs the qi of the liver meridian, it produces tension, which leads to increased heat. Boyle's law tells us that when pressure increases in any given volume, the temperature also rises, in the body as well as in laboratory experiments. Anger can produce internal pressure, which also converts to heat. The heat rises and increases, resulting in red face and eyes, a raised voice, headaches, and hypertension, which, in the long run, damages organs and exhausts vitality. Long-term tension can also stiffen the liver, reducing its ability to transform hormones, proteins, toxins, and emotions. During the premenstrual period, agitation can mount and migraine headaches, breast pain, irritability, and an overall feeling of malaise can develop.

But anger does not have to be negative and damaging to the body. When it is expressed directly and completely to release the liver pressure, it can be a beneficial force to help us overcome barriers and leave unhealthy relationships or work situations.

Several ideograms from the Chinese language describe this movement. The most common character, 氣, shows the movement of qi under pressure, like the weather. Another, 惱, depicts the heart and brain on fire. One symbol, 鯤, shows a fish transforming into a bird, breaking through the water and rising up in the air. This implies a violence proper to all beginnings: the force necessary to overcome resistance and to allow the birth process. Another ideogram, 怒, illustrates a heart and a woman under someone's hand, implying slave-like treatment and injustice. Anger can be beneficial and positive here; it is not damaging when it helps us recognize something inherently wrong and is used to break the bond holding the corruption in place.

To release suppressed anger, communicate your frustration about the situation that's angering you. Internal dialogue that merely justifies your point of view fuels the conflict. Feel inside to see if you are inspired to thoughts or actions that make you feel better. Would it help to talk to someone about it? Meditate about it? Journal about it? Stomp, cry, or scream? And, finally, when you have found a way to release, it will allow you to accept what remains, and from that place find compassion for yourself and others. Let everything else go.

When there is obsessive thought, qi is knotted

Obsessive thought is any negative thought, consideration, reflection, or form of attention that cycles around and around without producing some advancement. When it doesn't result in a beneficial shift in consciousness or inspiration to action, thought can become tangled, with no beginning and no end—a maze in which someone can get lost, dragging around personal troubles and the world's difficulties. This internal oppression becomes wedged, preventing qi from circulating properly and injuring the body's organs' ability to function.

When the heart, the empress of all our organ systems, falls prey to this internal angst and constant recollection, its natural outward movement becomes thwarted. It becomes caught up in its own image, like Narcissus, and can only think of itself. The self, discon-nected from its true nature, perceives only lack. The world, then, is not seen as a place of endlessly abundant glory and magnifi-cence, but merely as a means to serve the self and its insatiable needs. In this bound state, the heart loses its ability to love and a person loses her ability to be her true self. To move past the knot-ted state of obsessive thought, find the spark of the Divine within the highest aspect of the earth energies, which allows them to lift you toward your highest purpose and then move out into the world to express it. Living from the soul, which is outward, keeps you from the contracted state of living merely for self-fulfillment, which is a leftover immature perception from a life not purpose-fully lived. Your thoughts create your reality, but they don't create you. You are not your beliefs. You are so much more. You are an expression of incorruptible spirit.

When there is sadness, the qi disappears

Because the metal energies initiate tightening, creating an energy vortex within the chest, excessive sadness can become a vacuum, reducing qi and hindering its movement. To people in the depths of grief it may feel as though if they give in to it there will be no coming back—and there isn't. There is only going through and coming out on the other side.

Larry and Jessica found their twenty-one-year-old son in their room after he had killed himself. Nobody could ease their pain, and they found they had no choice but to go through it. And in doing so they discovered a depth in themselves and each other that they wouldn't have known if not for this loss. And this gift that they learned is something they can share with others in need of healing.

While we resist grief and loss like no other emotion because it reminds us of our mortality, we need to accept, experience, and let go to enable qi to flow. When we surrender to the pain of loss, sadness, and grief, we heal ourselves and emerge stronger than we were before.

When there is excessive elation, the qi becomes loose

Like all the other emotions, joy, too, can become excessive. When we overemphasize the importance of outside stimulation to make us happy, we can spend too much time seeking pleasure and excitement and lose the ability to know what makes us truly happy because we're not connecting to the inherent joy within. We trust less in internal cues and depend more on external consensus; in other words, we live from the outside in, rather than the inside out.

But when we find the joy within, we don't need to seek joy elsewhere. Because the heart houses our direct connection to the Divine, it provides us with a natural feeling of ecstasy that can be endlessly replenished and needs no outside stimulus. An open, balanced heart expresses joy, contentment, and gratitude for life. It lets us live in harmony with ourselves as well as the world around us. As the heart pumps blood throughout our body, the spirit pours love beyond the body and gives us a sense of oneness with the universe and the knowledge that we are part of Divine creation.

Barbara arrived at the retreat as sweet as she could be on the surface but angry and repressed inside. She made a fuss when anything wasn't to her liking and constantly complained to my staff, though she acted like an angel around me. When I worked with Barbara, I learned that she had been sexually abused as a small child and that the anger she still held inside over what had happened to her had seared her blood, not allowing it to flow. Her treatment plan consisted of expressing and releasing her anger and finding her real sexual identity. With time she was able to do this and became a counselor for abused women.

Equalizing Emotional Energies

Women don't heal through the accumulation of mental knowledge—they heal with their bodies. So when unexpressed or excessive emotions accumulate and obstruct qi, women need to move their bodies to express and release the emotions and reclaim their vitality. I use the following movement exercise to help women release obstructed emotions.

Flowing with the world

You may do the entire exercise at the same time or the relevant part when the particular emotion reveals itself to you. As you act out the movements, you may want to play music that helps you express the emotions. The process may evoke some difficult feelings, but if you are willing to trust that the discomfort will pass, your inner healer will resolve what no therapist can.

Remember that there is nothing wrong with any emotion, and it's not necessary or helpful to chastise yourself for how you're feeling at any moment—even if you feel you've lost ground and aren't feeling as joyful as you were. Your emotions are important, ever-fluctuating tools of self-evaluation and guidance, and as natural as breathing. But how you handle them makes all the difference to your health and well-being, so use these exercises to help keep the energy flowing.

When there is fear, lift the energies within from descent to ascent. When you notice fear in yourself, lie down on your side, with your knees and hips bent, curled up in a ball. Breathe deeply into your source as you consider how fear draws you in to protect yourself. Feel the sense of fear you have about anything in your life that makes you feel unsafe. Acknowledge the fear. Breathe into it. See it for what it is, and find your foundation of safety within. What can help you rise above the fear? Often, fear is rooted in not feeling deserving or in a feeling that someone is going to do something that will negatively impact your life. If this is so, look for ways to soothe yourself, remembering that well-being is your natural state. Know that when you stay balanced, then you stay aligned with the universe and nothing that happens can shake your Divine connection for long. Little by little, continuing to breathe deeply, bring yourself from this spineless, contracted fetal position into a strong upright stance.

When there is anger, let off steam. Wherever you feel internal tension, frustration, anger, or fury, breathe rapidly and shallowly into that part of your body. Then exhale forcefully. Shake out the anger. Yell it out. Scream it out. Stomp it out. Do whatever your anger inspires you to do until you have released all the built-up tension. Then allow yourself to collapse and feel for that place of pure compassion for yourself and the original source of your anger.

When there is obsessive thought, untie the knot of bound qi. Do you have discomfort in your belly, a gut reaction to stress? Bring all the neurons, the cables of tangled thought, to that spot deep inside your belly. Feel the tension condense into a tightly closed fist that tries to hold onto something that doesn't really exist. See the fist in your mind's eye and clench it even tighter. Then slowly open the fist, finger by finger, unclenching the hand and letting the tension go until it is just an open palm, receptive to nourishment and fresh new options.

When there is sadness, bring the qi back. With your arms folded over your chest, feel the loss, whatever it is. As you inhale, experiencing the pain and loneliness, tap with your fingertips over your breastbone to release the energy, then open your arms wide, exhale, and let them go. Let the part of you that is attached to grief expire with the breath as you open your arms. Then, when you feel the sense of release, exaggerate the exhalation. Feel the emptiness between the exhalation and the next inhalation and notice how your breath returns naturally, filling your lungs with acceptance and love. Receive the love that comes with the spirit of your breath.

When there is excessive excitement, reel in the qi. If you find that your quest for external fulfillment is causing you to lose touch with your body, bring it inside. Feel the loving spirit and send it to penetrate every cell in your body. Love yourself and forgive yourself, and forgive others as well. Through your blood and your spirit, feel the beat of your heart and the love it spreads. Send the river of love, unconditional and unrestricted, to the depth of your source, to the pure potential within you. Then invite all the other energies to join this powerful force to help you recognize your true self. Realize that you are overcoming the conditioning that has prevented you from reaching your highest state of being and, through love and compassion, feel the miracle that you are. Such connection can help slow down your activity to a pace that is balanced with stillness.

> *In the end these things matter the most:*
> *How well did you love? How fully did you love?*
> *How deeply did you learn to let go?*

> —THE BUDDHA

Secret 8:
Live "Vertically" Instead of "Horizontally"

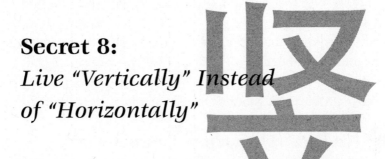

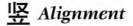 *Alignment*

*Jadelike purity has left a secret of freedom in the lower
   world:*
*Congeal the spirit in the lair of energy, and you'll sud-
   denly see*
*white snow flying in midsummer, the sun blazing in
   the water at midnight.*
Going along harmoniously, you roam in the heavens
Then return to absorb the virtues of the receptive.

—THE SECRET OF THE GOLDEN FLOWER

An ancient Taoist text, *The Secret of the Golden Flower*, describes the miraculous exchange between fire and water: when the fire of our spirit mingles with the depths of our source, the resulting power enables us to spiral upward and transcend the material world, to live on the plane of the phenomenal.

As discussed earlier, and illustrated in the horizontal-vertical grid, the horizontal plane is the "doing" plane, where source and spirit manifest through the material world: projects, work, family life, creativity, thought, word, and deed. The vertical plane is the plane of "being," where our Divine nature manifests, aligning itself with our highest spirit to let our radiance shine through.

The Vertical Conduit of Fire and Water

Water is the medium that joins heaven and earth. It rains down from the clouds and, through the power of the sun, evaporates from the earth to start the cycle over again. In the same way, water connects the lower body's energies with the fire of the upper body, joining our potential to our highest expression, enabling us to live our destiny.

The fire–water connection reveals itself most notably between the first menstrual period and the last. At menarche, the onset of menses, the heart brings blood and its life-giving spirit to the uterus, the "palace of the child," and endows it with the ability to bring forth life. At menopause, the end of menses, the uterus gives the gift of life back to the heart so that its love and wisdom can be shared with the world.

The channel of communication between the heart and the kidney essence, represented by the creative powers of the uterus, must be open for the spark of life to be ignited in any form. The void in the center of the heart and the void in the center of the uterus are the sources of women's strength and conduits to the universal process of creation. When obstructions exist, life energy can stagnate, but with proper attention and honoring, our inherent creativity can once again flow.

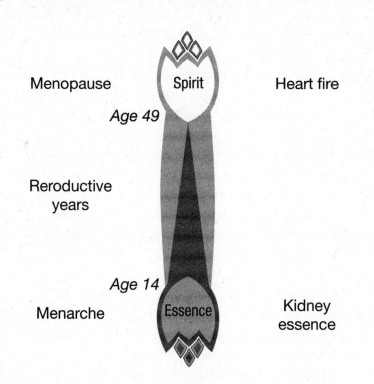

Menopause	Spirit	Heart fire
	Age 49	
Reroductive years		
	Age 14	
Menarche	Essence	Kidney essence

✽ The Maturation Process

According to the I Ching, seven is an auspicious number, and we can see its importance when we look at typical female maturation. Women typically mature in seven-year periods: In times when women were in touch with nature and themselves, most girls lost their baby teeth around age seven and started menstruating at age fourteen (the age today can be as young as the single digits). By twenty-one, their hormonal, reproductive, and musculoskeletal systems are developed and by twenty-eight their vital energy, blood, and organs are at peak condition. Then, at age thirty-five, women's skin begins to change; the complexion wanes, and hair color begins to fade around forty-two. Menstruation ceases around forty-nine (though today the average is closer to fifty-two) and the physique becomes more delicate.

The maturation process is revered by Eastern cultures because of the wisdom gained through experience. Women entering the revered state of menopause feel surges of heat as their fire energies shift upward to fuel their transition to the highest level of heart-centered wisdom. While many Western women resist menopause, matriarchal cultures see it as a time when women increase their power. In Chinese, there is no word for menopausal symptoms, because the process isn't resisted. The Chinese believe that heat or discomfort is natural and should be accepted—a rose does not resist the opening of its petals. According to this system, resistance disappears when you treasure nature's ability to allow you to unfold into your most radiant bloom.

But it takes tremendous energy to fuel this vital process. To enable your body to function at its best during menopause, I recommend eating a healthy diet, nourishing your source, and drinking additional water so the kidneys have an abundant supply. While this natural condition is not an illness and doesn't need to be "healed" per se, certain herbal blends (such as black cohosh and epimedium) and supplements (such as calcium, magnesium, and vitamin D) can help support the body as it experiences these changes. Though Western medicine is still undecided on the effectiveness of these natural therapies, many of them are supported by long histories of traditional use. Before trying these therapies or making changes to existing treatments, be sure to check with a naturopath or other health care professional who is knowledgeable about natural medicine to avoid interactions between supplements and medications.

🌸 The Dynamics of Fire and Water

Fire is the ultimate yang element: it is bright and moves upward and outward. But with enough fuel, fire can burn out of control, devouring everything in its path. The ego, like fire, can burn out of control when it feeds on itself too much, and become an insatiable flame.

Water is the ultimate yin element: when permitted, it goes deeper and deeper, always seeking darkness and depth. But water is also associated with fear, and can become a tool of the ego, supporting its false need to protect itself. Then the water element can approach the world as if everyone in it is its enemy, waiting to drain or pollute it.

Fire and water keep each other in check, as do their associated organs, the heart and the kidneys. The kidneys provide coolness, moisture, and nourishment to balance the heart's outward dynamic, but if there is conflict between the two, either of these elements can take control. When fire burns out of control because the kidneys are unable to cool and nourish properly, you may become restless and unfocused. You may also lose perspective because your emotions are erratic, or tend toward anxiety because your spirit has no nourishment or reason to come home to the heart. Conversely, when the water element is too abundant, it may put out the heart's fire. You may become depressed and begin to spiral down.

We in the West tend to favor light and brightness and reject everything that we consider dark and negative. We look for external happiness and elation and try to avoid being melancholy by covering up and ignoring negative feelings rather than using the information they give us to help us reach again for connection. We reject yin, or darkness, but it is yin that puts lightness into perspective. As we look to move to ever higher planes of vertical living, we need to accept all of ourselves, both the light and the dark, and know that no emotion is ever inappropriate. By learning to shine the light of our spirit on all that we have hidden from ourselves and from the world, it's possible to rise above the debris buried in our deepest caverns and find grace.

Rebalancing the Vertical Energies

Holding on rigidly to familiar horizontal energies—the consuming "doing" actions that gratify the ego—blocks women from reaching their spiritual potential. For optimum health and fulfillment, uncover and nurture three areas of vertical bodily energy: the lower abdomen, the midsection, and the chest and head. As explained in Chapter 1, the lowest area is the foundation of life, or source energy, that houses our innate talents and our ability to create and reproduce. The middle area, or soul energy, spreads horizontally across the center of the body and enables us to express ourselves to the world, through thought and emotions, words and deeds, and to receive expressions from others. The highest area, or spirit energy, connects us to our spirit and urges us to manifest our best selves and be unconditionally joyful.

Calm, happy lives result when the three energies are balanced vertically, but most women expend an overwhelming amount of their soul energy living horizontally, involved in too many external activities, obsessed with their thoughts, and not nurturing their core self and spirit. You know what it feels like to live this way—drained rather than vital and fulfilled.

In order to tune in to your inner vertical connection, your energies can be rebalanced by making lifestyle changes. These include setting and respecting boundaries that relate to all the things you do: eating healthful, whole, organic foods that won't stress your digestive and metabolic systems, and practicing breathing techniques that connect your spirit with your source.

Supporting your vertical growth has the added benefit of protecting health as your alignment helps reduce stress and thereby illness. While thousands of years ago the stress response was essential to survival, today we have neither the constant need to run for our lives nor to live a life dictated by the senses. Today we have the opportunity to live from spirit in a state of abundance.

Rising Above Obsessive Desires

While desires are natural, they can prevent movement up the vertical plane. They can keep you bound in a pattern of feeling deficient, then acting to satisfy cravings from a place of disempowerment, then wanting more because of increased desire but feeling even more powerless to achieve your desires.

When yearnings are aligned with the movement of your heart and are in harmony with your surroundings, they can heighten and add to your spiritual connection. But when you hold desires that feel enormously important but fearfully and frustratingly unattainable at the same time, you actually block their fulfillment—even the purest, most virtuous of desires can turn into a prison when you are so attached to an outcome that you lose connection with who you are and what you really want in life. For example, most people's desires are to be happy, spiritually enlightened, healthy, and so forth. All our yearning relates to that overriding desire somehow, but it's often easy for people to lose sight of the big picture and insist that it must happen through a particular relationship, job, or other goal. People in this position are like the archer who was overly attached to hitting his mark, about whom the Chinese philosopher Chuang Tzu once said, "The need to win drains him of his power."

Have you ever wanted a particular romantic relationship so much that your excessive longing blocked its happening and caused misery rather than fulfillment? Have you found that when you are able to stay open to any turn a relationship might take without needing a particular outcome, it unfolds much more harmoniously? The well-known example of women who desperately want a baby getting pregnant after they have adopted a child and released the focus on pregnancy is the perfect illustration of how obsession interferes with fulfillment.

Here are some examples of how unfulfilled desire can become obsessive:

Pure Desire	Attempt to Fulfill	Result
Baby is hungry.	Cry isn't answered.	Even food won't satisfy.
Teenage girl wants a boyfriend.	Girl focuses on a boy who isn't interested.	Girl becomes obsessed, feels inadequate, jealous of other women.
Woman wants a child.	No pregnancy ensues.	Woman must have a child at all costs, even at the expense of her relationship, feelings of self-worth.
Woman desires love from husband.	Husband is emotionally unavailable.	Woman has affair, satisfies lust but still craves love.

How can you avoid obsessive desire? Here is how the above examples might play out when the person does find fulfillment:

Pure Desire	Attempt to Fulfill	Result
Baby is hungry.	Cry is answered.	Food is very satisfying.
Teenage girl wants a boyfriend.	Continues to enjoy her own interests.	Retains her control over her happiness, attracts someone who sees this in her.
Woman wants a child.	May try to get pregnant but also spends time enjoying children of family friends, and her other creative interests.	Has regular, satisfying interactions with children and/or with her creative output, which makes her relaxed, happy, and more likely to conceive.
Woman desires love from husband.	Husband is emotionally unavailable.	Woman focuses on restoring her love for herself; husband is either attracted back to her from her lovely place of connection or she can clearly see that it's time to move on from him.

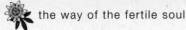

When trying to let go of an obsession that already has a strong hold over you, it can help to shift your focus away from the object or subject of your desire and remember that you get to choose whether you align with your desire or not. Let's look more closely at how that works with an unfulfilled wish to conceive (you may replace the word "child" with any other desired object; the same process applies):

1. You desire a child—purely.
2. Unfulfilled attempts to have a child lead to *resistance*—feelings of fear, anger, and deprivation. Spending time on negative thoughts—worry about not being able to get pregnant, jealousy over another woman's pregnancy—adds to this resistance, worry, stress, and a horizontal attempt to control your desires, which closes off the source (uterus) from the life-giving powers of the heart.

OR

3. *Pure* knowing that what is essential will come to you, in some form or another, as long as you pay attention to how you feel and stay open. This process actually opens the spirit-source axis, aligning you with the universe's ability to fulfill your desires.

Take time to meditate and spend time noticing and appreciating the many blessings of life, from the most commonplace (flushing toilets!) to the most personal (how your pet looks at you while getting stroked).

If you correct imbalances at Step 1, the longing will remain pure, undiluted by fears and frustrations, and there will be no resistance, or resistance will drop away. In the example above, in other words, if you try to catch yourself when you start to fall into insecure thoughts about having a child and instead focus on gratitude for all that you have rather than worry about what you don't, resistance will melt.

How you choose to respond to unfulfilled desires makes all the difference—not for the chances of your future fulfillment, but because it means you are living a happier life *right now*. If you stay in the precious moment and take care to align yourself with your source and spirit, your heart energies will stay open, allowing your qi and blood to flow smoothly. Practicing the breath exercise later in this chapter will help you more easily return to a state of calm.

The key to ensuring that a pure desire doesn't become tainted and lead to obsession lies in learning how to let your mind become still. Stillness, like water, reflects all that is, yet does not become the things reflected. Pure perception can happen only in stillness, after the waves of emotion have been calmed. When the energy of an emotion has been mastered, the meridians release it, like rivers leading out to the sea. There, in the current of life, joy is naturally felt and expressed. As the Confucian philosopher Xún Zi said,

> No one who pays undue attention to external objects can fail to feel anxiety in her mind. No woman whose behavior departs from true principles can fail to be endangered by external forces. No woman who is endangered by external forces can fail to feel terror in her mind.
>
> If the mind is full of anxiety and terror, then, though the mouth be crammed with delicious food it will not recognize the flavor, though the ear listens to the music of bells and drums it will not recognize the sound, though the eye lights upon embroidered patterns it will

not recognize their form, and though the body is clothed in warm, light garments and rests upon fine-woven mats it will feel no ease.

In such a case a woman may be confronted by all the loveliest things in the world and yet be unable to feel any gratification. Even if she should feel a moment's gratification, she could never completely take off her anxieties and fears. Hence, although she confronts all the loveliest things in the world, she is overwhelmed with worry, and although she enjoys all the benefits of the world, she knows only loss . . .

But if the mind is calm and at ease, then even beauties that are less than mediocre will gratify the eye, even sounds that are less than mediocre will gratify the ear. A meal of vegetables, a soup of boiled greens will gratify the mouth; robes of coarse cloth, shoes of coarse hemp will give ease to the body; a narrow room with rush blinds, a straw carpet and a table and mat will give comfort to the form. Hence, one may not be able to enjoy all the most beautiful things in the world, and yet she can still increase her joy . . . This is what it means to value the self and make other things work for you . . .

When you release a specific object of your desire through acceptance and surrender, and focus only on the larger desire of loving and caring for yourself, you will be fed by the earth's power of intention and transformed by wood into the unlimited abundance of the spirit. Entrusting the desire to nature's Divine grace will allow the Divine to see to the desire's fulfillment and open you to the creative power of the universe—love.

Reaching Your Highest Destiny

*In the depth of winter, I finally learned that within me
there lay an invincible summer.*

—ALBERT CAMUS

As you've seen, throughout the book I've written about the spiral journey up through three levels of existence—source, soul, and spirit—that enable you to live joyfully, express your true nature, and reach your highest destiny. In Chinese, the three levels are called *jing, qi,* and *shen,* and are thought of as anchoring, aligning, and adapting in *The Way of The Fertile Soul.*

❀ **Anchoring**—Source energies anchor you to your innate self: the gifts, talents, genetics, and constitution you are born with. By anchoring yourself to your own true nature—the good and bad, the light and dark—you develop and grow, as long as you remain flexible enough to change in response to your changing world.

❀ **Aligning**—When properly anchored, your heart's spirit aligns you to your purpose and dreams. Aligning allows you to learn how to best make use of your talents, what to let into your life, and how to live passionately from your spirit. With alignment comes the ability to make your own music rather than dance to someone else's tune and yet live in harmony with the world.

❀ **Adapting**—When aligned, you can respond authentically to your environment and life circumstances. Interactions become pure, unhindered by selfish motives, and possibilities abound, resulting in thought, reflection, and action inspired by alignment. When you have adapted to your world, you become serene and undisturbed, because you have tapped into your inner wisdom, which has nothing to do with schooling, intelligence, compliance, or societal expectations. You know intuitively what to do and feel supported by the universe, whose laws you now live in harmony with. Your soul expresses the Divine in accordance with an anchored source and an aligned spirit.

This state of being contains unadulterated promise—hope in its purest form. Having hope is not wishing for material things or what you think will make you happier, like being skinnier or having a certain partner. Having hope is being open to whatever wonderful gifts life brings you, trusting that it will unfold

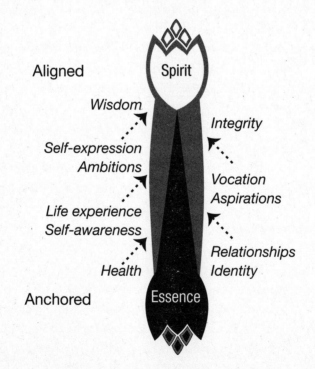

perfectly. Even if you experience something that feels like a "setback"—a miscarriage, losing a job, not qualifying for a grant or a loan to go to school or start a business—nothing that has happened in the past need impact your future if you can keep honing your ability to return to that open state of possibility.

When you live vertically, the energies of the horizontal plane support your vertical ascent. The vertical energies urge you to fulfill your highest potential rather than squandering your promise in material pursuits. At the apex of your existence you live having "turned the light around," a Taoist expression for turning your energy inward and giving birth to your true self.

To support your quest to live vertically, regularly practice the following meditation, which uses the senses of hearing and seeing to shine the spiritual light within.

Meditation to Turn the Light Around

Begin by sitting comfortably and taking some long, deep breaths. Bring your awareness behind the center of your eyes. Feel a connection between that point and the center of your head where the energies of your ears converge. In Taoist tradition, if you listen when there is no sound, what you hear is the universe, the sound of creation. So listen to the soundlessness of your breath and feel the power of the silence within. Notice how you can receive the information your senses provide you without interpretation or judgment; if you find such thoughts creeping in, acknowledge them and then let them go and return attention to your breath.

See with a deeper vision; hear the deep silence; smell the clear openness. Savor the taste of pleasure itself. Feel the gentle touch of your own life. Let your senses draw in the depths of your surroundings like the leaves of a tree turning to the sun, simply attracting the nectar of life. Open wider to receive more, with absolutely no effort.

Connect with the heavenly bodies, the sun and stars, and feel the connection between these fire energies and your heart. Open your heart as you draw in more warmth, and then breathe it down to your uterus to connect with the spark of the Divine within. Allow your womb to receive the heart's warmth and to open up to its tremendous healing power. Drink in the warmth and become aware of any blockages preventing the reception of your love. If you discover any barriers, acknowledge them. Thank them for their message. Then release what is blocking your love and bring down more spirit. Open up to as much love as you can take, receiving the abundance of spirit into the void of your uterus, letting unlimited love unite with your Divine source. Your deepest sense of wisdom and deep knowing reside within your depths.

Continue bringing the warm fire energies of the sun and stars down and letting them merge with the well within your own source, until you feel that the circuit has been completed deep within. Let the energies swirl, envisioning the red fire energies joining with the blue water energies to become one conjoined energy, purple at the center, red at the top, and blue at the bottom. This energy represents your true purpose, the reason you were born. Draw these energies into your core, and go completely into your center, into the depth of your being, as if all of the fire energies above and water energies below are merging as sap in your core.

Pull your attention back toward your spine, further away from the exterior, away from the branches and leaves of your external life situation, and allow them to fall to the ground and drop away. Turn your awareness within to your trunk, and bring it down into the depths of your own roots—from the spine to your sacrum to your feet, connected to the ground, where minerals are absorbed and merge with the stillness within the frozen ground, where life waits patiently to be coaxed into a new spring. As you send your own energy down into the earth, let yourself become as still as winter.

When you feel the connection with the ground, know that you will receive whatever it is you need from Mother Earth, and let the fire of the spirit's sunlight ignite the spark of the Divine fire deep within down through your roots. Awaken to visualize yourself turning toward the new dawn of the East, and turning away to release all that you wish to let rest in the West, as you spiral vertically to awaken into the summer of possibilities, reaching your most joyful goal. You are a wonder, and you hold the secrets of all creation within you—from the kernel of life hidden beneath the frozen earth, to a budding flower, to an exploding star.

> *I died a mineral, and became a plant.*
> *I died a plant, and rose an animal.*
> *I died an animal and I was a man.*
> *Why should I fear? When was I less by dying?*

> —RUMI

Secret 9:
Reenergize Yourself by Repatterning

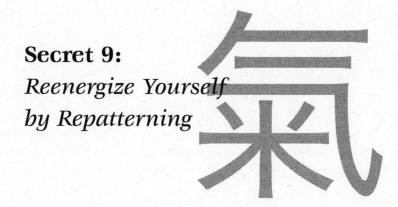

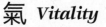 **Vitality**

You must learn to be still in the midst of activity and to be vibrantly alive in repose.

— MAHATMA GANDHI

Because we live in a yang-dominated society that values ambition and measurable success over stillness and introspection, we favor the mind and its external projections rather than nurturing and living from our yin energies. Repatterning can help restore balance in women who have lost theirs.

Even patterns that have served us well can become our undoing if we don't let them go when we have outgrown them. For example, a woman may develop a healthy pattern of intolerance to an oppressive situation, and that resistance will allow her to find a way out (leaving a failed marriage, for example). If this experience empowers her to trust her natural inclinations and feel the universe's support, then she will reach a new place from which to spontaneously try creative solutions to other new challenges. If, insecure about herself, she feels the world is hostile, she clings to the resistance that helped her before. However, after the situation changes, the resistance may turn into frustration, anger, bitterness, or resentment and start to fester, producing a toxic inner state.

After learning to release emotions and address each of the energy tendencies in the body, the next step is repatterning harmful past conditioning. You have the tools to transform yourself into whatever it is you wish to become. Stressful patterns of the past will dissolve as you recreate yourself in accordance with nature and discover new, energizing patterns.

Just as a seed is transformed by the dark underground forces to joyfully emerge as a sprout, your transformation takes place in your depths. The following meditation exercises will enable you to reach the Mysterious Mother—that Divine feminine potential that has been waiting within you—and uncover hidden difficulties, emerging transformed and renewed.

Inviting the Winds of Change

Chinese medicine incorporates the concept of an internal wind, which not only accounts for internal shaking movements like twitches but also initiates the alchemical transformation process, which can be seen when someone in a deep meditative state begins to shake. This tremendous force gives power from within just as the earth restructures itself through earthquakes;

the internal winds of change come from awareness that things inside need to change.

To start your transformation, invite the purification process by allowing your internal winds to blow and paying no attention to the external winds in your environment. Instead of blaming outside forces, let your internal wind help you reclaim your personal power. When you know you have control over the way you react to any situation, you can take full responsibility for all you do, instead of avoiding, denying, or resisting reality in harmful ways, such as escaping through addictive behaviors or substances.

In the depths of your being, water will transform you as the immense geyser of your true self erupts. As Lao Tzu tells us, you will "be like water, and go to the places loathed by [wo]men . . . deep beyond knowing . . . still enough to awaken slowly into life . . . and you'll wear away into completion."

To go to your depths and release the powerful winds of change within you, perform the following exercise regularly, being gentle with yourself throughout and remembering that there are no wrong responses. This is the complete process of inner alchemy, the pieces of which we have explored up to this point. Create a comfortable and sacred meditation space in your home; when your world becomes sacred, without and within, the Divine will step in to help you reach your goals. The more you practice, the more you will become acquainted with your purifying inner depths.

Journey Through the Body's Inner Universe

This exercise is best performed in a chair, with your bare feet planted on the ground and your head lifted. Breathe in through your nose, following the breath past your heart, lowering your diaphragm to allow your belly to stick out as you inhale and to sink naturally as you exhale. The deeper you breathe, the lower your energy level will drop.

Start by bringing your attention to the center of the bottom of your feet, the source of the bubbling spring. Root yourself to the earth and feel the warmth coming up to you from the magma in the center of the earth. Follow this energy up, through your legs, your sacrum, spine, neck, and head. Then bring your awareness to the top of your head and draw in healing energy from the sun, which melts you from your head down. Feel your head melt into your ears and face and neck and your neck muscles melt into your shoulders. Let your shoulders melt. When you feel completely relaxed, begin the following exercise.

Step 1: Harvest your inner potential

Bring your awareness to just below your navel, where your most powerful energy lives, in the lower chamber of essence where the uterus resides. Feel yourself breathing in and out through your chamber, as though your belly button is doing the breathing. Fill your belly and pelvis with the qi of life. Then extend the channel that runs horizontally along your hip bones like a belt and feel it as a shield protecting your body.

Step 2: Activate your qi

The microcosmic breath

Breathe in through your nose, placing your tongue on the roof of your mouth. Draw a golden cord of light through the microcosmic orbit: begin at the perineum, between your vaginal and anal openings, and draw the breath energy up to your navel and chest to connect with the energetic point between your eyebrows and up to your crown. Release the exhalation down your neck, spine, and tailbone, scooping up air with the next inhalation. Continue this form of breathing throughout the exercise.

The internal smile
This smile is one you don't simply make with your lips. This is a cellular smile that enlivens your organs with appreciation. Like when you gaze at a loved one, send love and attention to each of your organs to encourage them to function optimally and help you find peace within.

Step 3: Heal
If you encounter a blockage as you do this part of the exercise, allow yourself to feel it and move through it. To refine the pain into a source of healing, connect with and regulate each of the energy elements and its organ system through quiet reflection.

The kidneys
Breathe into your source with the intention of opening yourself up to learn who you are at your core. As you breathe in, feel your kidneys in your lower back, tucked beneath your bottom ribs. Bring the warmth of your heart's fire down past your kidneys and into your chamber of essence to connect with the life-giving energies of the uterus.

Feel into the depths of your being, your essence, your makeup, the home of your DNA, the person you are meant to be. Deep within, deeper than what you do in life, deeper than the fear of not being enough, lies your original Divine gift. You consist of all that came before you, in a unique patterning of your life. Your DNA contains messages passed down from your ancestors that are always available to you. Think about places in your life that are working, and about what you would like to see more or less of. Think about what you have covered up and need to expose to yourself. Acknowledge the latter gently and compassionately—life can be hard, and all of us need to withdraw at times. Breathe into your fear, see it for what it is, see that it has no power over you, then release it from the safety and security of your own source. Feel the spark of the Divine and listen to your inner voice, which will always tell you truths.

The liver

The large, expansive liver, which is located under your right rib cage, branches out to purify, transform, and rid the body of all that is not helpful or useful. Bring your attention to your liver and visualize the color green—sprouting, growing, expanding, and generating. Think of a tiny acorn becoming a towering oak and the energy that requires.

Now connect with your own power and reflect on whether there are any inner directives you haven't carried out. Do you have pain stuck inside that festers as anger or some other emotion? Have certain barriers prevented your growth? Are there situations you feel have caused you to stagnate? Do unfulfilled desires bind you up inside? Remember that denying what you find inside will not allow a solution to emerge. Locate any tightness and recognize how and where the frustration has produced tension in your body.

Then, feel how the trapped tension wants to get out. Breathe quickly and shallowly around it—hyperventilating—until it is bursting with the attention of your own qi. Then, let the tension rise to the surface of your body, moving upward and outward, and release it deliberately, even forcefully: flail your arms, scream, stomp—whatever it takes to get the tension out. Next, turn your appreciation inward to the liver's ability to transform and the strength it provides you to achieve your goals. Connect with your deepest vision, your innermost dreams. See them clearly. When you connect with the power of your imagination, you unleash the power of inner transformation and allow your dreams to become reality. Breathe your own healing breath into your liver and feel the pressure release as the energy flows freely. Be grateful to your liver for all it does for you.

The spleen
The earth energies of the spleen, stomach, and pancreas allow you to take in what you need to nourish yourself and release the rest through the bowels. The earth energies also represent the thought process, which can be ineffective when cluttered by constant thinking that doesn't produce action. Ask yourself if your thought process is clear and unhindered or if it is weakened by worry. Do you obsess about what you don't have?

To unclutter your thoughts, bring your awareness to your solar plexus, midway between your breastbone and your belly button, where the earth energies are located. Focus on your center. Consider whether you are able to let in things that are good for you and nourish your body and soul and if you're able to release things that don't support you. Breathe deeply into the middle of your abdomen, the home of your spleen and stomach, and focus on the breath. Fill your empty abdomen with earth energies and let them untie the knots of worry and obsessive thought. Release the thoughts and open up your center to let fresh, healthy nourishment in. Allow an internal vacancy that can be filled with fresh options.

Take some deep, cleansing breaths and experience the state of openness and receptivity. Let thoughts come and then let them go, like clouds passing through an open sky. In this state, like a magnet, you draw to yourself the focus of your intention.

The lungs

Healthy lung energies represent the face you show the world. They enable you to both form bonds with others and relinquish those that are no longer in line with your highest purpose. The lungs symbolize the solidified physical self at one end of the spectrum, rigid and confined, and the ability to decay, dissolve, and be reborn at the other end. Hildegard von Bingen said, "The soul is for the body as the sap is for the tree," and the soul energies unfold as the tree unfolds its gestalt. The lungs signify the return to the innermost self, the way a tree provides sap to its roots in the winter.

To activate the lung energies, bring your awareness to the center of your chest. Feel the inward pull as your chest expands on the inhalation. Feel yourself being breathed, in and out, through no effort on your part as you breathe in the aroma of life. Bring your awareness to how your breath moves inward, representing the contraction of sorrow from your initial separation from the Divine. Follow the movement to the center of your chest and then feel its contraction of individuation as it meets the heart's outpouring of love. This is the place where your separate self ends and you become one with the spirit of existence.

Notice how your breath continues through you—to benefit from it, all you have to do is receive it. Feel the acceptance and embrace the breath of life. Feel the clear, crisp, cool white energy rush in and out with each breath you take. Feel the courage you receive by accepting and surrendering to every breath. Release each breath fully, opening yourself up to receive again. Exhale fully, relinquishing everything that has kept you from expressing your highest good.

The heart

The heart, the empress of the body, mind, and spirit, circulates pure, unconditional love through your body and connects your spirit with the spirit of the universe. The heart energies are passionate and warm, expansive and limitless, and, when the heart is healthy, they radiate peace, love, and joy.

To activate these energies, bring your awareness to the center of your chest. Feel the warmth of your heart and see how deep inside you can feel its beat. Now, expand the feeling and see how far you can project your heart's love outward into the cosmos. Continue to do this for as long as you can. As you project love, you honor yourself with the power of the spirit.

Step 4: Liberate

From tapping into your unobstructed healing energies within, your body becomes more open, enabling you to become a channel for creation.

To open yourself to receive your heart's warmth and your body's healing energies, go back to the center of your being, the chamber of essence. Picture your earliest memory of yourself as a baby. Breathe deeply into your source and meditate on the face of that child. See in her eyes the full potential of who she was created to be—before she received any messages about who she *should* be. This is your true self. Her essence contains your innate gifts and her Divine spark is your Divine spark. She is the inner driver of your subconscious mind.

Now, bring those gifts and dreams into your present-day self. Integrate the two parts of yourself and feel the life and the love. Receive. Be grateful. Acknowledge who you are. As the river accepts the raindrops and the ocean welcomes the rivers that flow to it, it is your nature to receive, for you are a channel of creation. Realize that you are a miracle and that, by staying true to your true nature, you can live your greatest dream.

Tina, a retreat participant, describes her journey through the inner universe:

> Then began one of the most profound experiences of my life. It was so intense that it seemed to go to the very core of my being, my very life force. Suddenly, I was lying next to everyone in this circle and people were all around me, but despite this I felt the deep reality of how alone each of us is. As single souls we enter the world and as single souls we die—the realization of this was so powerful. I understood that no one can be what I am or experience what I am feeling except for me, that each of us, although we exist alongside each other, has a personal and unique journey.
>
> The power of that feeling was overwhelming—as if a curtain had been removed from between my normal daily life and the profound reality of life. The truth was laid bare. It was at that moment that I thought that in this lonely life the most precious gifts might not be granted to me. I think for the first time ever I really came face to face with my fears, the fears I kept so tightly locked away. At that point I welled up with tears so intense they were unstoppable. Sobs shook my body, rising from deep in the base of my stomach.
>
> But then a sort of withdrawal started to take place. An image formed as I faced my fears. Above me was a circle, a Source, and behind me the world and all that I hold dear. Over my shoulder I could see and sense the green world, my dear, dear angelic husband, the

dreams I had for my life. Amazingly, despite the fact that my hopes and my dear one was behind me, I was focused on the circle above. I kept repeating to the circle, "Bring me closer to you, let me come closer to you, take me to you."

The intensity of my pleas grew to equal the intensity of my sobs and seemed to come from the same place, deep at the bottom of my stomach. But then I became overwhelmed by the realization that despite all my yearning, I didn't need anything or anyone—not even my husband, who is such a treasure to me. I gradually realized, like some sort of gift being handed to me, that the only true source of peace, comfort, and joy was the Source above me. Everything else was a diversion, even an illusion. It was as if I was moving towards a universal center and that all earthly things were behind me. Only my desire to move closer to the source remained.

As I kept pleading to move closer, I realized that I wanted nothing else, just that. Everything that I had yearned for and that I had and cherished seemed insignificant. Then, in the depth of the experience I began to fear that perhaps I actually wanted to die, but I realized that this couldn't be because my heart was full of love and longing for the Source above me.

Afterwards I remembered a saying by the prophet of Islam, Muhammad: "Die before you die." I wondered if this was what I had felt. The experience had the feel of passing into a different realm and through different and intense emotions, in some way a death-like experience. It was an abandonment of everything that I held dear, which all seemed minor, almost illusory, compared to the Source. Through that understanding and that experience I found my unity, my strength, my peace within. I became the healer I was looking for.

Mandala Making

The final step in savoring the inner journey is one of my favorite retreat projects: mandala making. Put on soft music, take a piece of paper, and draw a large circle on it, nearly touching the edges. Then draw a smaller circle in the middle of it that represents the earth. Then separate the large circle into the four quadrants of the other elements, like the illustration below.

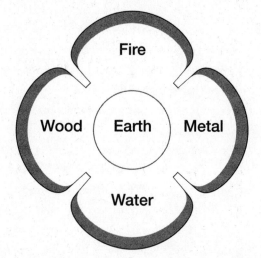

On a copy of the circle above, use paints, markers, pencils, or chalk to draw a pictorial representation of what you felt and saw on your inner journey, to help you integrate your meditation into the creative aspect of your body and mind. Display your mandala on your wall or sacred space afterwards to remind you of your growth and change. Make a mandala each time you feel yourself growing and changing. The artistic process can access answers from deep within and show you the way.

Painting is just another way of keeping a diary.

—PABLO PICASSO

Secret 10:
Match Your External Actions to Your Internal Blueprint

行 *Embodiment*

*If you want to know your past, look to your present
  conditions.*
*If you want to know your future, look to your present
  actions.*

— Buddhist saying on Karma

Just as energy flows through our bodies, it also flows through our brains. And just as bodily energy can become blocked and stagnate, so can the energy in the mind. Because we create our reality out of our thoughts, imbalanced brain energy and negative thought patterns can obstruct our ability to create the reality we dream of.

The mind controls the body's responses and actions through positive thoughts, the placebo (literally, "I shall please") effect, and negative thoughts, the nocebo ("I shall harm") effect. Those who believe they are going to recover from an illness usually do, and those who think they are going to die are more likely to. Women who believe they are weak become sickly. People who complain they never get a break never do. Those who fear they may be infertile usually become so. Over and over, the body plays out the story that the mind creates. Releasing negative thoughts and beliefs associated with the lower thought patterns of fear, anger, worry, and grief and looking instead for evidence of love, well-being, abundance, and joy open women to experience unimpeded possibility.

From the first nine secrets you learned to rebalance your body's energies to reach your highest level and find the calm within. Now we will integrate that knowledge with the workings of your mind for complete well-being.

Early on in my career I treated many people with depressive disorders and other mental disturbances. Working with them made me understand that psychological discord, which shows up as chemical imbalances in the lab, is not actually disease but rather energetic imbalances that manifest as mental disruption. These deep imbalances result from ignoring our true nature and resisting the flow of the universe.

Rachel was a pharmacist who had an apothecary at her daily disposal. As patients refilled their anxiolytic and antidepressant prescriptions, Rachel realized that she, too, was anxious and depressed. She started helping herself to the abundant promises of "feel good" drugs and eventually became addicted to Xanax. She also lost her job and her pharmacy license.

Reaching this state was actually the beginning of Rachel's real healing, because it forced her to look at her life. When she did that, she realized that she had become a pharmacist to prove to her alcoholic father that she was smart and worthy and wouldn't succumb to his vices. But her perceived antidote had become her poison.

Eventually, Rachel went into therapy. She also followed the ten secrets to deal with the emotions behind her depression. As her brain cleared and her body and spirit healed, she discovered her inner truth and realized that becoming a naturopathic physician was her true purpose—which she did.

Traditional Chinese medicine does not ascribe a particular organ system to brain function. Instead, the brain is viewed as an extension of the kidneys, a kind of information processor generated by the kidneys' essence; the spinal column and the brain stem are also considered extensions of the kidneys. However, *thoughts* and the functioning of the brain are ascribed to the five energy elements, each of which is associated with a particular area of the brain and its functions. Each element also has a special association with memory and higher intelligence. As with the physical and emotional beings, the workings of our own mind provide a blueprint of reality that links us to the elements in nature. Note that the representation of the brain is actually a mirror image of outer life.

All of the brain's functional areas are connected by a network of corpus callossum fibers that allows us to do multiple mental and physical tasks simultaneously. Women who have raised their consciousness and found wisdom and insight actually increase the functioning of the corpus callossum fibers and have access to all domains at once. Researchers have found that the brain function of those who meditate regularly has more action in the higher-functioning frontal lobe than the lower-functioning brain structures. The upper center of the frontal lobe lights up with the state of intention and sets up the rest of our brain's priority by what we choose to attend to.

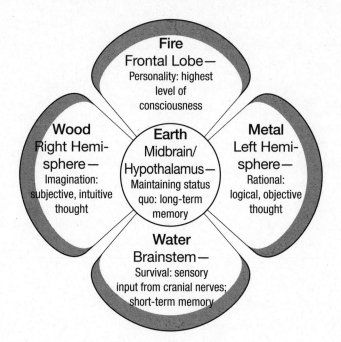

In later years, changing hormone levels can alter brain function. There are changes in the ability to concentrate, and people often experience emotional ups and downs. Then, as we move further toward death, we lose some short-term memory. Long-term memory function remains, but our senses start to fail us, as well as certain functions that are tied to survival. As difficult as these changes can be, it makes sense that, as we are pulled closer to spirit, our worldly survival functions decrease, helping us to let go of the world. Western society is obsessed with finding the fountain of youth through external means, but there are people everywhere quietly living long, fruitful lives, who radiate inner health and happiness with increasing power until they joyfully leave their bodies. Decline doesn't mean decay. The process of aging isn't something to be resisted. With the lessening of the five senses, the emphasis becomes less about the form of this manifestation. As our outer vision begins to weaken, our inner vision sharpens. The letting go of the physical is a natural process of releasing to spirit.

Like the migratory birds that have the iron-based chemical magnetite in their brains that helps them navigate, our human brains guide us through life like a sophisticated compass. And like the qi gong masters, yogis, and others who exercise their ability to tap into nature, we, too, can increase our ability to navigate well by rebalancing the energy elements of the mind.

Instead of fighting the situation and keeping yourself trapped in that pattern, it's possible to uncover the real cause of the problem and correct the imbalance through meditation and reflection.

Rebalancing the Brain's Energy

Traditional Chinese medicine approaches mental disturbance the same way it approaches disturbance in any of the organ systems: locate the origin of the problem, address the root imbalance, and let it fall away. For example, consider a situation you've been in that you didn't like but couldn't change. Perhaps you resisted it and the resistance became frustration, which then fueled anger. Because you were taught not to express anger, the unexpressed anger produced inner tension, making you feel stuck, a form of depression.

Each energy element can be addressed to enable the brain to return to smooth energy functioning and to synchronize the energies of the left and right brain. Each element has a lower and higher energy function. One keeps us stuck, and one liberates us to higher functioning. When we focus our actions on the superior function, we reinforce the elevated brain functions. This prepares us to match our external actions to our inner blueprint.

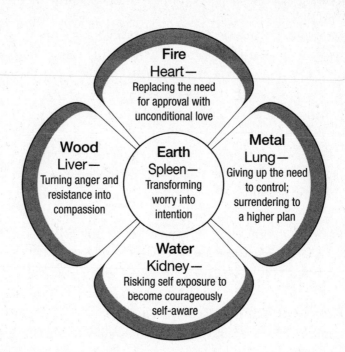

Fire
Heart—
Replacing the need
for approval with
unconditional love

Wood
Liver—
Turning anger and
resistance into
compassion

Earth
Spleen—
Transforming
worry into
intention

Metal
Lung—
Giving up the need
to control;
surrendering to
a higher plan

Water
Kidney—
Risking self exposure to
become courageously
self-aware

The water energies

If you are constantly in survival mode and feel that fear and self-preservation are controlling your life, your water energies are out of balance. In the same way that water seeks to fill every crevice, fear floods every part of your being.

When I talk about fear at my Fertile Soul retreats, I ask the women to pretend they are surrounded by a pack of hungry tigers. When I ask them what they will do, the usual replies are "Climb a tree" and "Run for my life." The best answer, however, is "Stop pretending."

Because most of our fears are unfounded, habitual reactions, the remedy for fear is to see the situation for what it is. Does it actually represent a threat? Sit quietly, evaluate the situation, and shine the light of awareness within to find your courage and strength. Remind yourself of your abilities to take care of yourself, and reach for the unlimited, universal love in your core. By bringing your awareness to the chamber of essence and breathing deeply, you'll not only reduce the output of adrenal hormones that is fueling your panic but you'll access your innate wisdom and begin to heal.

Much of our fear is inspired by worry that we're going to lose something we have (our health, our children, our security) or fail to gain something we want (affluence, a long life, a child)—desire giving rise to trepidation. Another source of worry is the thought that we will be found out—that we've done something terrible that we can't acknowledge ourselves, let alone share with others. Much of our fear, however, is really of our own making. When you look in every nook and cranny, you may find that your secret is really not so terrible. I was amazed to find that many of my own secrets, which seemed so shameful to me in private, were trivial once they were revealed. Fear is usually more horrifying than the thing that is feared.

The wood energies
When anger and resistance are getting the better of you, you don't have access to the higher mental function of imagination, so you can't match your external actions to your internal blueprint—which is necessary in order to turn your dreams into your new reality. The key to unblocking access to the right hemisphere of your brain, where imagination lives, is to physically release anger and let compassion in by following your angry impulses until you feel some relief. You might hit a pillow. Stomp on the ground. Drive into the country or take a walk by yourself. You might feel like going to a place where you can

scream and cry loudly and out of control, until you get all the anger out of your body.

When the fury has gone, look for the place of compassion within, where you find release and forgiveness. Tune in to your higher energy as you breathe into your liver. Smile a cellular smile. Be kind to yourself and let energy flow throughout your entire body. Then release the right side of your brain and let it fulfill its potential. Unleash your creativity and imagination, the inner artist that we all have, so that your actions match the wishes of your heart.

The earth energies

Worry, concern, overthinking, anxiety, and obsessing muck up thought processes and keep us from turning our intentions into actions. When we're so knotted up with worry, it's hard to trust enough to let go. But as you practice letting go, staying open, and expecting things to work out, the world will rearrange to match your outlook.

Start by bringing your awareness to the moment. When you walk, focus your attention on the sensation of your feet meeting the ground. When you prepare dinner, place your awareness in your hands as you chop vegetables, observing, smelling, feeling, and appreciating the plants that are about to nourish you. When you are fully focused on your activity, focus on your sense of being: how it feels to be in your body, how the breeze feels on your skin, how your energy feels inside your tissues, how your inner spaciousness is expanding. Connecting with what you're doing and how you're feeling stimulates the right side of the brain, where creativity and imagination live, and enables you to turn intentions into actions.

To lessen the pressure when you're overly worried and are not yet able to refocus your attention, do something pleasurable like reading a light, fun novel, watching a favorite, funny movie, or looking at a pleasing piece of art or other things of beauty. When possible, avoid noisy filler like television commercials that are designed to manipulate people.

You can also do something—anything—creative: gardening, cooking, painting, drawing, knitting. Playing with whatever medium you choose is an easy way to align your energy.

The metal energies

The metal energies are associated with the left side of the brain—the orderly, logical, rational control center. While this part of the brain allows you to organize and make sense of your world, trying to control too much will keep you from connecting with the creative side of your being. It will also give you the illusion that you can control the world, which can then lock you into grief, sadness, and eventual depression and collapse when you realize you can't.

Trying to control other people, places, things, or situations is futile—but we can change our attitudes toward those things in order to take control of ourselves and how we feel. This requires relaxing the rigid control of the left side of the brain in order to release, expand, loosen up, break free, open up wide, and shake up your world. To do this, practice doing something silly or out of character for you. Make up a song. Try a new craft or hobby—even if it's something that scares you.

The fire energies

As you learned in earlier chapters, your spirit wants to express itself so that it joyfully flows upward and outward, as is its nature.

This happens when your fire energies are unobstructed and unhindered by thoughts of worry, anger, sorrow, and fear. According to neurobiology, humans cannot be simultaneously protective and expansive. When in fight-or-flight mode, overriding concern with self-preservation diminishes your growth and life experience. However, as you practice what you've learned in this book, you allow your heart energies to spiral up and open your fertile soul into its inherent expansive state. As you practice the exercises, you will find the gift of inner stillness where the fountain of love begins to flow. Decide to find this love and uncover the wonders of creation.

To strengthen the fire energies, connect with the beauty of nature: a flower unfolding, a tree reaching its branches toward the sky. Embrace all of creation and meditate on it. Savor life and its design, including your own. Let the love in your own heart grow so that it can open the window in your mind and work in harmony with all of creation.

Right brain–left brain functioning

The corpus callossum fibers connect the lobes of your brain, allowing you to access both right- and left-brain function simultaneously. Try these exercises to expand the smooth working of this synchronization:

1. Regularly practice this qi gong exercise: create a figure eight with your hands, moving them back and forth in the sign of infinity, crossing them at the midline.
2. Dance, using steps in which you cross one leg over the other, bringing your right leg to the left side and your left leg to the right side.
3. Wear your watch on the opposite wrist from your usual.
4. Write in a journal daily to express your innermost self. Try using your nondominant hand and allow your writing

to be messy and expressive. Keep lists of things that bring you joy: loved ones, favorite memories, future exeriences that you anticipate with pleasure.

These kinds of exercises help the mind expand. Such expansion is not limited by intelligence or education, but comes from intention, attention, and practice. To replace old patterns with new ones it's important to reinforce your new chosen ways of being and thinking with daily practice.

Exercise also helps to rebalance brain energy and lift mood. Studies have shown that daily walking and swimming can increase levels of the brain's feel-good chemicals, such as serotonin, norepinephrine, and endorphins. It also helps to talk to friends and counselors—let life be your therapy. Try also to keep sugar and refined carbohydrates out of your diet. Eat oily fish such as mackerel, halibut, sardines, salmon, and tuna and consume the abundance of organic, nutrient-rich fruits and vegetables.

Enabling the expression of love

When your external actions match your internal blueprint, you flow with the universe and the way things are. You don't resist, you let go of what causes stress, and you adjust your attitude rather than trying to adjust the world.

When you operate at a higher level, negative lower-level reactivity falls away. Many patients I've treated have had respiratory allergies, food sensitivities, and negative environmental reactions that disappeared when they stopped resisting and began accepting. My own damaging reactive processes, including arthritis, ulcers, irritable bowel syndrome, and migraine headaches, stopped manifesting after I began to live according to The Way.

When you accept life on life's terms, you allow the laws of the universe to support you. Rather than living a draining struggle, you live effortlessly and selflessly, with love flowing like a river through your heart.

> *Love is a force in you that enables you to give other things. It is the motivating power. It enables you to give strength and power and freedom and peace to another person. It is not a result; it is a cause. It is not a product; it produces. It is a power, like money or steam or electricity...*
>
> —Anne Morrow Lindbergh

Like any flowing body of energy, love must have an outlet so that it doesn't become stagnant and more love can be received. Many women send out their love by mothering children, organizations, projects, individuals, and communities. Mother Teresa is an example of this highest state of selfless loving.

But when the expression of love becomes obstructed, inner joy stagnates and you may begin to feel that your life has no purpose. Many women who feel this way turn to plastic surgeons, new romantic relationships, or a multitude of material projects, but these kinds of reactions do not enable love to flow.

Following *The Way of the Fertile Soul* will keep you on a path of joy and enlightenment that the Taoist sages set forth when the world was their guide. As William Wordsworth said, "Come forth into the light of things; let nature be your teacher." While some of nature's changes along the way might seem violent or mystifying, remember that nature has a plan for you and will guide your body, mind, and spirit. So feel the fear of change, but do it anyway.

Daphne, a beautiful Italian woman I helped at a recent Fertile Soul retreat in Ireland, expressed this magical secret poignantly: "I have existed for forty years with all the tools I needed for life on earth. But nobody ever provided me with the instruction manual on *how* to use these tools until now. Now I know how to live." By following *The Way of the Fertile Soul*, Daphne came into the light and took to heart the old Zen saying: "You cannot tread the Path before you become the Path yourself." Daphne found and became her path, the path that had always been there waiting for her to follow it. She opened a nursery school to be around the freshness of young children.

The ancient wisdom of the I Ching says that all things go through cycles of change, driven by the opposition of yin and yang. When a cycle rises and reaches its apogee, it then transforms and descends into its polar opposite. In this way, all of us go on a circular journey that spirals back to higher levels of ourselves, and those who are wise engage in meditation and self-cultivation to become more sensitive to the inherent movements of this natural cycle. Enlightened people do not see hard luck as tragedy: they see it as a learning opportunity, a chance for change. They are forever grateful for every situation and welcome both positive and negative experiences equally. They wear the world as a loose garment, with the ability to act appropriately in all settings. And as they become aware of the cycles of life they let go of the burden of the suffering self and feel lifted by the universe.

If you look back at the many meaningful events in your life, I believe you will see that all along, life has been giving you clues to lead you toward your best destiny. Don't dwell on the past or try to predict the future, but do think of every moment as a critical juncture in which you can become more sensitive and more receptive to your inner strength and wisdom and to the pointers and subtle signs that nature is sending to you. Then, with reverence, humility, and service to others, you can reach higher levels of being and live the Divine life.

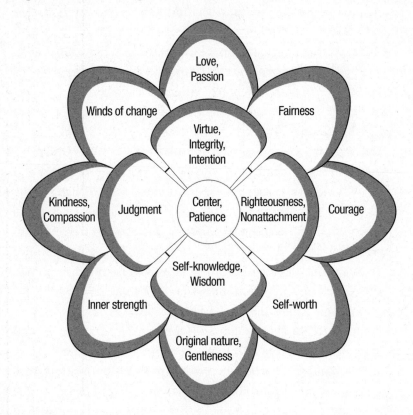

In the above illustration, the blossom shows how deep awareness and solution-based action uplift us. In your personal life, for example, if a problem with your kidney system manifests in a hormonal imbalance—lack of libido, for instance—you can look at your deepest level of being, your original nature, and ask yourself with gentleness and compassion which inner needs are not being fulfilled. If you experience shortness of breath (which involves the lung or metal energies), you can look at areas in your life in which you lack courage. If you have a great deal of anger (which involves the liver or wood energies), you may need to exercise the solutions that directly impact wood: using inner strength and judgment to change the situation, or adopting an attitude of compassion to accept it.

You can receive all of life's answers by using this model. Think of the center as the place where all the elements are balanced and where you go to wait for the correct answers to be revealed. There are times to act and times to be inactive, to wait instead of moving hastily in a way that is not appropriate to the situation. When you don't know what is appropriate, the answer—always—is to become still and turn to your center for guidance. Through meditation, put yourself into the background, beyond the difficulty, away from the problem and its talons of control, to find your truth.

"Feng shui-ing" your actions

The Chinese have a concept called *ling*, 靈, which means *divine state*. The Chinese character for ling is composed of raindrops falling from heaven, while two priestesses performing a ritual dance to effect changes in nature. The Taoist sages used rituals that raised their vibratory level to create changes in the world, which they called alchemy. The rituals and practices of *The Way of the Fertile Soul* can similarly connect the spark of the Divine within you to the spirit of the Divine without, which will align you with the will of heaven and create the appropriate context through which change can occur.

I call these practices or actions "feng shui-ing" your life. You may already be familiar with feng shui, the ancient Chinese practice for maximizing the eight vital areas, or *baguas*, of your living environment. The practices I've developed align with those principles, working to attract positive life energy and keep it flowing and unblocked, so that you can live comfortably and naturally.

Just as there are eight vital areas in your home, there are eight vital energy areas of your life (see the diagram below) that form a circular path and are as important as the vital energy areas of your environment. The love area of your home is as important as the love actions in your life and the money area of

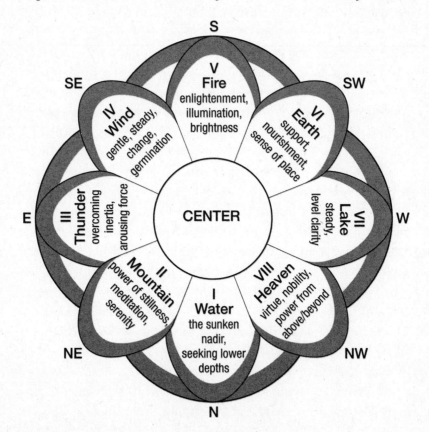

your home is as important as your inner sense of value and worth. And just as you use feng shui to align furniture and spaces in your home for maximum energy flow and effect, we will use it here to align your actions for the most positive outcome, based on your individual characteristics.

When you place yourself in the empty center—your true self; nothing added, nothing taken away, looking out at the world around you—you will see its goodness and how its elements care for you. Note that when you are in the center, you face the direction where the sun shines most brightly (the south), with the energies of emergence (the sunrise) to your left and the energies of return (sunset) to your right. Your water or source energies are to the north, behind you, forming your base of support.

The numbers, going clockwise from Water to Heaven, represent the trigrams presented in the octagonal bagua life compass presented in the I Ching. When life isn't moving along easily, and we have relationship, work life, or personal difficulties, the path might look very different (see illustration on next page).

When you feel difficulty in any of these areas in your life, don't reach for a quick external solution; contemplate the higher energy for this same area. For example, when I have difficulty in a particular area, before I take any action, I go to the circular meditation garden in my backyard. I face the direction of the particular bagua so its answer can be revealed. For example, if I am feeling rigid and uptight about something, I sit and meditate facing southeast and focus on the winds of change, seeing what needs to be changed in me and my response. To use this technique, try to consider the root of whatever is bothering you. Does it feel more about fear or impatience? Are you feeling like a victim? Or powerless? Are those feelings coming from an

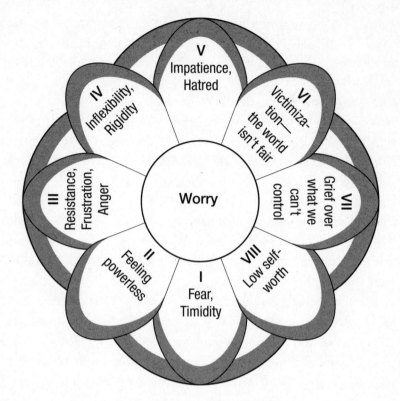

actual threat, or just worry over something not wanted? In other words, something that's not real?

When you have located the area of blocked energy in your life, you can learn the answer to the problem by using the Path of Answers below to shift your energetic response to the situation. Move along the path, reflect on the problem, and then find the inner wisdom that leads you to the answer to your predicament. As Albert Einstein once said, "We can't solve problems by using the same kind of thinking we used when we created them."

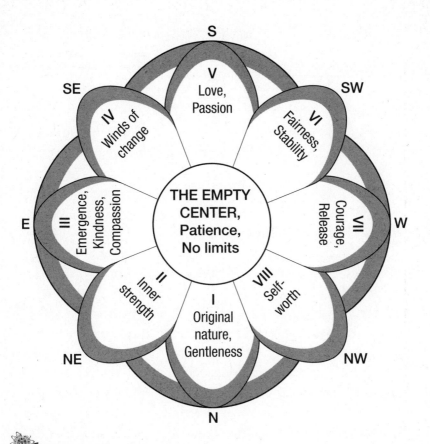

The Path of Answers

This method could be considered the Tao of troubleshooting problem areas in your life circumstances. It is not a salve simply to make you feel better, or an outer directive derived from experience. The Path of Answers leads you inward toward your own wisdom, reminding you that you already have all the answers you are seeking. Find the area that most represents the problem you have in your life, and compare it with the solution. This takes you from the lower contracted state to a state where your energy is freed to find the solution within. This brings us to the Chinese concept of 无未, *wu wei*: doing without doing. There is nothing to force; only reflect, find the inner stillness, and let your own answers emerge.

Fear

You may remember that fear and timidity are symptoms of blocked water energies. When you feel paralyzed by fear, you need to go deep within to where your water element resides and find those aspects of yourself that are scaring you. The depth is called the nadir, the lowest point, opposite the zenith on a celestial body. Instead of turning away from the fear or trying to hide it, as most people tend to do, the answer is to go within and, with gentleness, find your eternal source of strength. That eternal source will provide you with what you need to know and enable you to live from your true nature. (See Point I on the three charts, beginning on page 192, to see how fear, water, and gentleness relate.) When my life goes through changes and I begin to experience fear of what my life will look like in the unknown, I meditate within, look at what I'm really afraid of (which is often simply fear of the unknown), and gently remind myself of my original nature—that I have all I need. No change need have power over me.

Powerlessness

Where do you feel weak or timid? It's possible to realign feelings of powerlessness if you are living according to other people's dictates, rather than your own. You have within you what you need to reclaim your power—you have a mountain of stability and the strength of a volcano.

Mountains are unmoving, strong, proud, and still. When you align yourself with the powerful forces of nature, you will find your true strength and the power of the mountain. To align your-self, be still like a mountain. Visualize yourself on a towering mountain peak, viewing the world objectively and understand-ing that some barriers must be acknowledged (for example, a sixty-year-old woman can't start a biological family). When you are ready to descend back into your surroundings, bring the power of the mountain with you. You are not powerless. (See Point II on the three charts to see how powerlessness, moun-tains, and inner strength relate.)

Frustration and anger

The loud clamor of thunder is representative of the force required to overcome the inner resistance that builds to frustration and anger. Thunder shakes, agitates, and upsets the torpor of inaction that can fester within and turn against you. Where do you need to take action? Where do you need the power of thunder to shake up what isn't working? Find your power and then balance it with compassion, which, like the rising sun, comes from a place of kindness and allows change. Compassion and kindness will enable you to find your inner voice, which cannot be squelched by the actions of others, and to overcome what needs to be changed within yourself or in your world. (See Point III on the three charts to see how frustration, thunder, and compassion relate.)

Rigidity

In what areas of your life do you feel inflexible, where you could use a little more suppleness? A position at work or a stiff relationship? Rigid trees can be toppled by a strong wind, but flexible trees such as hollow bamboo can flow and move with it. Because we cannot change or stop the wind, it's essential to move with the inevitable changes that blow through our lives.

Consider where you need to be flexible and when you should raise the sails of your soul to catch life's power and go where it is taking you. Observe the power of the wind as it turns a windmill, lifts a kite, carries a bird, pushes a sailboat, gently ruffles your hair, rolls and rocks a tumbleweed. Then let yourself move with your personal winds of change and purification as you remain rooted and stable deep within the ground. (See Point IV on the three charts to see how rigidity, wind, and change relate.)

Impatience and hatred

Is impatience, lack of joy, or hatred keeping you from shining in the world? Is there a person, institution, or political situation toward which you feel intolerance, annoyance, or hatred? If so, forgiveness is the key, burning away these lower, stagnant energies so that the light of your spirit and inner divinity can radiate through. Fire and its brilliant powers burn away hatred and let warmth and joy spread upward and outward, letting your highest nature gleam with love. Fire and passion, however, can burn out of control, so it's important to tame them with restraint and channel them into appropriate arenas. Bask in the warmth of your love and use it to ignite the spirit of others, but don't send your passion unchecked into the world. (See Point V on the three charts to see how hatred, fire, and love relate.)

Feeling victimized

When you feel as though you're a victim of your circumstances and life isn't fair, you need a good dose of Mother Earth. Open yourself to receive the earth's nourishment and support and allow yourself to grow in her rich soil, fed by her lakes and rivers, mighty and calm. Be fair like Mother Earth, who has no favorites and does not provide according to who is most deserving. Give because it is your nature and ask for nothing in return. Be patient, kind, and fair, and accept yourself for who you are. (See Point VI on the three charts to see how victimization, earth, and fairness relate.)

Grief

Life cannot be controlled, and this can cause grief and sadness when something happens that we don't want. One of my patients was still in deep grief eighteen years after her mother died, thinking of her and crying many times each day, which kept her from living life fully. The solution is to recognize and accept the disorder and fractal qualities of life, surrender to them, and move on with courage and purpose. Then, like a lake whose mud settles to the bottom, calm will descend, and clarity will be revealed.

Lakes, like people, teem with life and abundance, but both also contain chaos, decay, and death. The lake represents the paradox of life and death and shows us how surrendering to whatever the weather brings, whether calm or storm, is how we find peace. Waves come and go whether we approve of them or not, and they cannot be resisted; they can only be released.

Like a lake that freezes in winter and thaws in summer, life changes. Even if your life seems organized and controlled, there is strength in recognizing that it is constantly moving and that the depth below the calm exterior is always churning. Courageously accept life's motion and understand that it results in goodness, joy, and harmony when you surrender to its sacred geometry. (See Point VII on the three charts to see how grief, lakes, and courage relate.)

Low self-worth

Difficult situations may trigger feelings of low self-worth. Many of us have felt worthless because of something we've done or because other people have told us we're worthless, but true self-worth doesn't come from what you do, whom you align yourself with, or how you appear. It comes from who you are—and you are the gem of the universe. You are a kiss from the galaxies, a nebula aligned in a double helix, a manifestation of heaven who contains the power of creation. When you feel worthless and low, remember that you are part of the cosmos and contain the nobility of the stars. You are worthy simply because you exist. (See Point VIII on the three charts to see how low self-worth, heaven, and self-worth relate.)

You may want to copy these diagrams and put them up on your wall or carry them with you in your handbag. If you can't find the answer to your difficulty in any of the eight ways described here, go to the empty center found in the diagram on page 192 and meditate patiently until the solution reveals itself to you. For example, if you feel out of control but can't find your answer in the wisdom of the lake, return to your center and look out toward the other seven solutions. Perhaps you need the inner strength of the mountain more than you need the clarity of the lake. Perhaps you need the enlightenment of love or the support of the earth. See which solution fits by asking yourself which qualities you can magnify to give yourself inner strength and peace. When you return to the stillness within and view the world objectively, nature will provide you with everything you need.

May the sun bring you new energy by day,
May the moon softly restore you by night,

May the rain wash away your worries,
May the breeze blow new strength into your being,
May you walk gently through the world and know its
beauty all the days of your life.

—APACHE BLESSING

3

*Keeping the Balance:
Easy Everyday Ways to
Stay at Your Creative Best*

继 *Continue*

免 *Freedom from Disease*

*Returning to the root is called tranquility,
Tranquility is returning to the inevitable unfolding of things,
Returning to the inevitable unfolding of things is called constancy,
And to understand constancy is enlightenment.*

— Tao te Ching

When you accept what is, you open up to the universe. When you accept what is, you stop fighting to impose your will. Instead, you surrender—but surrendering doesn't mean you stop trying. You keep trying, and sometimes failing, but you try without swimming against the current. You act and move forward and do the next right thing, but you do it as part of the flow of the immense current of life. You let go of outcomes and, as the *Bhagavad Gita*, the book of wisdom, says, you do your duty but without attachment and reach your ultimate truth without anxiety. From this place, any creative endeavor is open to you: having a child, starting a business, or deepening a favorite artistic, physical, or mental practice.

Happiness and Healing

I hope the ideas and practices in this book help you reconnect with your true nature and live in harmony with the universe. When you find your own source of healing, you can help the people you love to reconnect with their own source of healing as well.

I have treated thousands of women and men, many of whom were diagnosed with all sorts of "incurable" diseases, but when they tapped into their internal healer, they transformed—body, mind, and spirit. They surrendered and became aligned, creating an opening for new life, and that new life came—not from desperation but because they remembered their inherent well-being and allowed it to flow in.

That same process applies to all true healing. When you rise above the level at which the particular disharmony exists, and keep the vibration of your body, mind, and spirit elevated, the disease can no longer manifest. When the elements are aligned, you open up to let the creative force of life shine through. The elements in the diagrams aren't shown in perfectly straight alignment, because they are in constant movement. This is an ever-changing, dynamic process; the movement itself is what allows you to spiral upward. You never get to the place where wood is fully aligned between fire and earth because it is the movement of the ethereal soul of wood itself that propels us upward. The metal—the corporeal soul—is a constant, ongoing

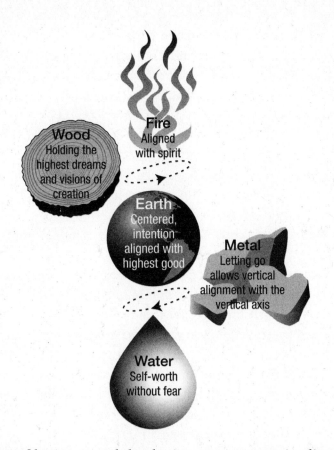

process of letting go and that letting-go process again aligns us with earth's intention and water's self-knowledge. It's a constant striving process—but it's not about doing. The movement of metal between the axis of earth pivots to bring us into alignment between earth and water. The movement of wood pivots around the axis of the earth toward fire, keeping us in a constant state of dynamic movement.

All of the previous chapters have described how to reach that higher level: to live from your spirit rather than from fear; to find balance; to listen to what your body, mind, and spirit are teaching you; to have emotional freedom; to live vertically rather than on the "doing" plane. By regularly allowing yourself to be still, to breathe deeply, and to seek your inner joy, you will become increasingly connected to your source and easily identify imbalances and put them right. You now know that you need not become a product of negative history. You understand how to live your life so that your activities support you rather than drain you dry. When you abide by the rules for being, there are no limits to what you can achieve.

Nurturing Your Creative Spirit

Before closing, this chapter will cover some tools to help you maintain a joyous connection to the source of all creative inspiration. Here are some everyday reminders:

- *Give yourself the gift of time.* The busiest, most successful, and happiest people I know make it a priority to take time for themselves every day. I meditate at least a half hour every day and I recommend that you do the same. Do not wait until everything else is done before you try to find time to meditate. Take time for yourself first. I promise you'll reap enormous benefits.

- *Pay attention to your inner world.* Connect with your breath—while you're cooking or driving to a board meeting or to work, anytime, anywhere—until it becomes something you do all the time. When you find yourself feeling anything but joy, breathe and focus on something that makes you happy to help you realign.

- *Recognize and love the Divine within you.* To continue to transcend your horizontal energies, you need to take care of your spirit so that it can support you at your highest level and enable you to face the world with strength, grace, and love. For each thought you hold, action you take, or difficulty you face, ask yourself the question: Does this nourish my soul or my ego?

In addition to these alignment tools, if you find yourself slipping back into unhealthy habits, as it is so easy to do, these three simple "body scans" will help you build your internal power. In each of these, honor your deepest self by allowing whatever comes up to be okay. It's not helpful to be disappointed with yourself for not feeling happy all the time. Remember that your emotions are natural reactions that provide invaluable information to help you adjust your energies and regain your balance.

If people can constantly be pure and still, then
heaven and earth will return to their places.

— Lao Tzu

Morning, Midday, and Evening Body Scans

Body scans are a useful tool for helping you identify distractions that might be muddying up your connection to the source of creative power. Try to use these three simple self-evaluation tools every day. They will help you understand what your body is telling you and what you need to do to reach greater well-being and fully express yourself. Performing these exercises each day will build your internal power and supply an energy bank from which you can always draw. When you live in this way, you approach all activities with the same joyous attention, and every interaction with others and with your own creations becomes an opportunity for growth and exchange.

When in this flow, you are always inspired to do the right thing at the right time, and you can tell whether it's the right thing by *how it feels to you—and only to you*. As soon as you factor in other people's opinions you won't be able to accurately understand your relationship to it.

Morning body scan

Start the day by sitting or lying quietly and connecting with the inherent joy of being alive. Take a moment to appreciate simple pleasures, such as a warm, comfortable house or dear pet. Relive pleasant memories and consider things you are looking forward to. Then tune in to your body and ask yourself what it is telling you today. Are you experiencing any physical discomfort? Listen to its message. Then consider what you need to do, right now, to give your body the attention it is asking of you. Take that message with you and let your inner voice guide you to release the discomfort and work through its message throughout the day. What are you inspired to do?

Midday soul scan

Begin by eating a mindful lunch. Feed your body and soul with what you really need, not just what your taste buds desire. If you indulge in a small decadent treat, savor it and know that it will nurture that part of you that deserves pleasure. After you eat, turn your awareness within, if only briefly. Discover which emotions are predominant in you today and think about what they are telling you. If you have negative emotions that you haven't expressed appropriately, decide what you are going to do to bring this reaction into alignment with your inner self. Tell someone safe? Journal about it? Let it go and focus instead on something rewarding?

Evening spirit scan

In the evening, think back on the day. Think of ways you expressed your highest self during the day. Reflect on actions that you performed with a sense of purpose. Think about whether or not your heart expressed its true desires and if your spirit will therefore find rest that night. Think about how much you have loved, both yourself and others. If you haven't met your own desired goal, know that tomorrow will give you another day to love a little more. And be compassionate and gentle with yourself. Allow the rest to come as you tune in to the song of your own heart and let it become your ever-present lullaby.

Creative exercises

If the daily scans tell you that certain energies are out of alignment, revisit the questionnaires in Chapter 2. Answer them again and determine which of your energies are obstructed. Then read through the information again and do the exercises in the appropriate chapter. If your emotions seem scattered, low, or out of control, check which energy needs to be aligned from the information in Secret 7. Focus on your current creative endeavor—whatever gives you pleasure. Keep a dream journal and become aware of themes that emerge through your dreams. Create something every day, not to make more stuff but to express yourself fully. Create a new dance, a new menu, a new way of looking at your life and those in it.

Expand the Moment

Every moment of every day, try to expand the moment you're in, enlarging your focus on whatever it is you are doing or not doing. Then drop into the background, away from whatever is demanding your attention, and let it take care of itself as you take care of yourself. Feel the energy behind what you're doing, then take that energy and bring it into everything you do.

Periodically check to see if you're living vertically—if your thoughts and actions are supporting your highest good. If you don't feel they are, work through the repatterning practices in Secret 9 to find equanimity. If you feel confused, read through the eight solutions provided in Secret 10 to find the answers nature offers to help you match your inner wisdom to your external actions.

And at any time, you can try to connect with the spark of creativity within your source. Marvel at it and feel how it

The Creative Process

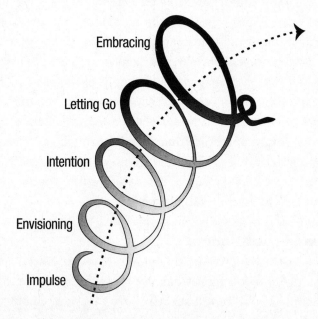

Embracing

Letting Go

Intention

Envisioning

Impulse

transforms all of life. Let yourself envision whatever it is you wish to create or become. Set your intention and let your actions support your vision, and let go so the universe can supply you with the abundance you were meant to receive. Remain centered and feel the love that's always there, waiting to be embraced.

Continuing on The Way of The Fertile Soul

As your energies spiral upward, unencumbered, people and circumstances that don't support your highest good will fall away. As you rise above your past difficulties and see that you created them and that you can let them go, you set yourself free. Little by little, you will return to balance and experience freedom, just like Keiko, who told me:

> After learning and practicing the ten secrets, exploring what life could look like began to seem intriguing rather than frightening. A feeling of peace began to emerge and it seemed possible to live life to the fullest and in the present moment. What is became fascinating. I found joy in the strangest places as well as the knowledge that I could and would be OK. Now I no longer hold back. I do things I am passionate about, spontaneously and randomly, and I savor every moment. I listen to and acknowledge my inner voice and I try to give back to others. I see possibilities everywhere and I feel gratitude for the gift of this perspective.

As you continue on your path, enjoying the expansion of your spirit in the endless array of creative endeavors, the tools and techniques in this book will support you. Embrace the creative

life force that shines through and allow the Mysterious Mother
to perform her magic as you soar higher and higher.

The Valley Spirit never dies.
It is named the Mysterious Female.
And the Doorway of the Mysterious Female is
the base from which Heaven and Earth sprang.
It is there within us all the while;
draw upon it as you will, it never runs dry.

—Tao Te Ching

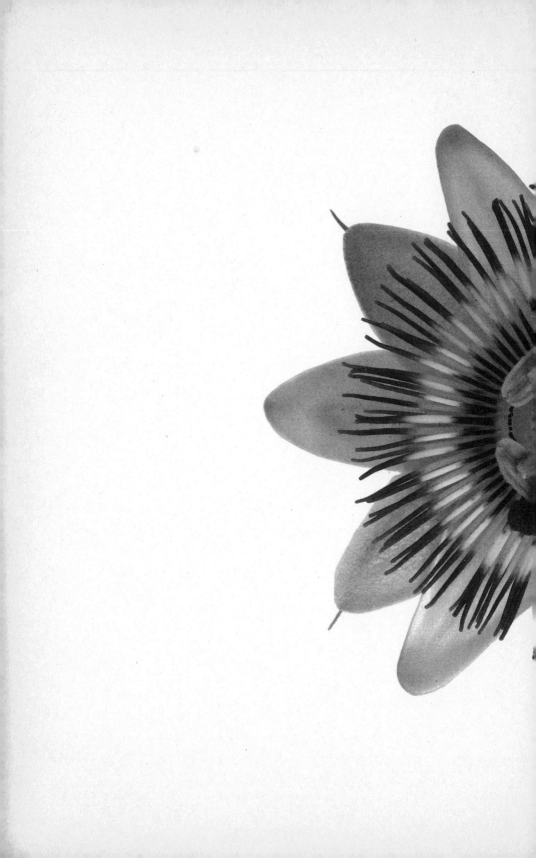

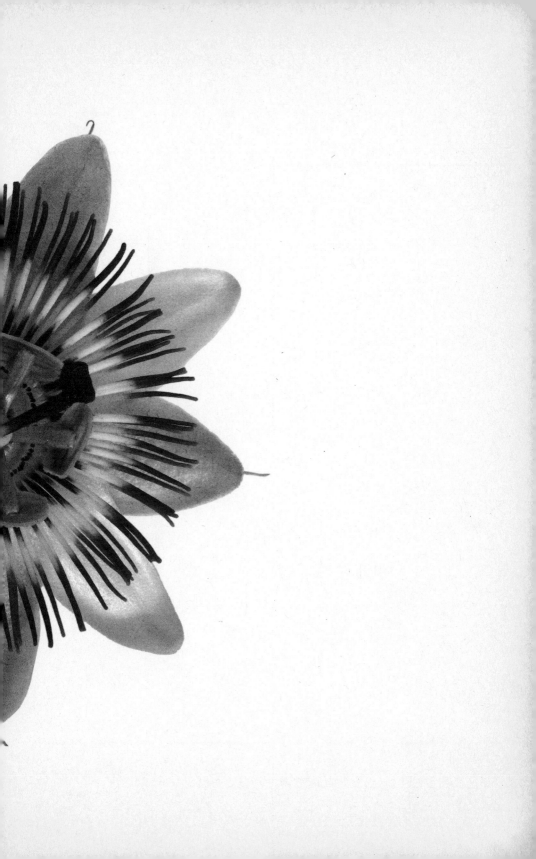